PREVENTION'S GUIDE TO
LOOKING FIT & FABULOUS

at Forty-Plus

by

Donna Lawson

Rodale Press, Emmaus, Pennsylvania

Printed in the United States of America.

Book Design by Anita G. Patterson
Illustrations by Susan Rosenberger

Library of Congress Cataloging-in-Publication Data

Lawson, Donna.
    Prevention's guide to looking fit & fabulous at forty plus.

    Includes index.
    1. Beauty, Personal. 2. Middle aged women—Health and hygiene.   3. Physical fitness for women.
I. Title.
RA778.L42   1987   646.7'042   86-26315
ISBN 0-87857-650-9   hardcover
ISBN 0-87857-651-7   paperback

2 4 6 8 10 9 7 5 3 1   hardcover
2 4 6 8 10 9 7 5 3 1   paperback

To Porky from Petunia,
to my "little sisters," Terry and Cheryl,
and to my friend
of 40-plus years, Diane Lund,
with love.

CONTENTS

Chapter 1
EATING RIGHT AT 40 PLUS

Crash diets are not the way to go when you want safe and lasting weight control. Here are some practical measures that will help you to achieve your goal. You will see why your body frame is a good indicator of what your weight should be, and how eating certain types of foods can help in reaching your own optimal weight level. Your mood can be affected by what you eat and so can your memory. The right food choices can help you to fight osteoporosis and cancer, too. The Turn-Back-the-Clock Diet (including menus for 21 days) shows you how to incorporate the foods that are best for you in your meals every day.

Chapter 2
ANTI-AGING EXERCISES

We all need some vigorous physical activity to keep our bodies from turning into blubber and our attitudes from turning into "old." Several over-40 women tell about their favorite exercise and what it does for them. Exercise will help to improve health and reverse many aspects of aging. Have a pre-exercise physical examination, choose the form of exercise that is best for you—and get started!

Chapter 7

SEX, SLEEP, SCENT & OTHER REJUVENATORS 191

Don't miss out on any of the experiences in life that can keep you feeling young and vital. For many women over 40 and past menopause, sex was never better, so take advantage of it as a sublime avenue to stress relief as well as the fulfillment of your romantic fantasies. Keep yourself feeling on top of life by getting good and sufficient sleep. Use any nondrug sleep inducer you need—from a comfortable mattress to a soothing cup of herbal tea—to do the trick. Use scent to please yourself as well as to attract others. Try making your own fragrances to soak in as you pamper yourself with luxurious baths. Surround yourself with people you enjoy, people who bring you up not pull you down. Go for the belly laugh. Build a good support system of family and friends. Keep your perspective about what really counts in your life.

Chapter 8

MENOPAUSE: MYTHS & REALITIES 221

Some women sail through menopause, and a relative few have a tougher time with this perfectly natural transition into a new phase of life. But all women get through it one way or another. Don't make it a problem if it isn't one. What really happens to your body at menopause? Hot flashes are explained along with the pros and cons of estrogen replacement therapy. Learn how to fight against osteoporosis, the ailment so common to postmenopausal women.

Chapter 9

FLEXING YOUR MENTAL MUSCLE 241

Just because a woman is past 40 doesn't mean that her brain automatically turns to mush. In fact, the mental stimulation at this age can be as good or better than ever before. But it calls for reaching out to new people and working at old friendships, setting new goals, and taking some risks. Insist on testing yourself with new challenges!

Chapter 10

FIT & FABULOUS FOREVER 255

All of the improvements have been made; now maintain the momentum. Here is a plan for setting your life up in a way that allows time for taking good care of yourself— a good diet, regular exercise, proper hair and skin care, good grooming, a little self-indulgence, and a lot of mental stimulation. You can do it all, and you can have it all!

INDEX 265

ACKNOWLEDGMENTS

Thanks especially to Sue Nirenberg, and to Molly McGrath, Jan Alexander, and Deborah Kirk for their help in putting this book together; to Molly (once more), Jeanne Conlon, and Abigail Thomas for "going to bat" for me and "getting made over"; to photographer Carl Doney for his patience, professionalism, and hard work; to Celeste Smith and Jenna Zark for lots of typing and photocopying; to my editor Charlie Gerras and to Camille Bucci, a whole lot of gratitude for their untiring efforts, encouragement, and understanding; to Sharon Faelten of Prevention Health Books for valuable suggestions; and to my agent Liz Darhansoff for her loyalty and support for how many years now.

INTRODUCTION:
TAKE ON A NEW CHALLENGE

What you have here is more than a beauty and fitness book. What you have here is a challenge. Remember challenges: We met them with relish in our twenties and thirties. Then 40 came and we hit a plateau. Our outlook became flabby along with our waistlines.

My friend Betty hit her plateau at 39, a year short of the mark. She said she was forgetting about her weight. She was middle-aged, and middle-aged women were supposed to be matronly. So she put away her bikini and put on weight.

I was appalled. "Betty," I said, "how can you be middle-aged? I'm not and I'm a year older than you."

That same year, a late bloomer, I fell in love with a man my age who had a teenage son and daughter. We got married and, love notwithstanding, he began to sound like my friend Betty. "Boy, wasn't it great when you could do this and that?" he'd say. I'd reply: "I don't know what you mean. I *do* do this and that."

Then something happened. Perhaps it was living with teenagers for the first time. They do have a way of placing you in a certain slot in time. "You mean you really saw the Beatles?" or, "You were alive in the 50s? Wow!" can make you feel like an old fossil.

Before I knew it, I started wearing my husband's old Lacoste shirts and invested in sensible shoes—matronly stuff. What did it matter? My bones began to ache and soon I had flab where my upper arms used to be.

Then Betty came around again. She was all decked out and thin on top of it. "I got tired of this matronly business," she said. "What happened to you?"

I took that to be a challenge. The next day, I skipped the double-double chocolate chip for Tofutti (128 calories), bought barbells and sexy underwear, and sent my husband's old Lacostes to Good Will.

Ten, 20, 50 lifts a day—my upper arms got tighter. Stretch, reach, stretch. My bones stopped aching. I lost weight. I even had a discernible bloom in my cheeks. No doubt the lifting, stretching, and running had a lot to do with it. But, it was more than that. It was my recharged attitude. I had moved off the plateau. I had met the challenge. And looking the way I was looking, it *was* a challenge.

In May of this year, I was 49. According to a recent article in the *New York Times,* if it were 1900, I'd probably be dead at my age. Now, I'd better be prepared to live to 90, says a friend whose field is gerontology. My friend told me, "We're living longer and at 70, you might find yourself with a couple of decades to go with nothing to do."

Women our age are lucky. Because we will soon be the majority of the population, there is great interest in us. Science is on our side. And so far the prognosis is good. With a correct diet, we're told, we stand a better chance of curbing the diseases that prey on older women: osteoporosis, breast cancer, and heart disease. Exercise, we've learned, will help us ward off bone loss, arthritis, and atherosclerosis (hardening of the arteries).

Not only that but diet and exercise are creating a lot of sexy grandmas; flexible women with small waists and tight thighs.

At my corner newsstand not long ago, I sneaked a look at *Playboy.* There she was, Terry Moore, a centerfold at 55. No one really knows how she got that way. She didn't say.

But, the very fact we have a 55-year-old woman posing as a pinup is news. When auto mechanics have a middle-aged woman posted on their walls, we know "prime time" has arrived.

We *are* getting fashionable. Shirley MacLaine kicked her heels up on Broadway at 50. Sophia Loren, 50, and Catherine Deneuve at 40 promote moisturizers and perfume on TV. Lena Horne is over 65. Then there is champion swimmer Donna de Varona, who anchored ABC's coverage of the Olympics in 1985, and yes, indeed, Joan Baez, who has gray hair like you and I.

It's easy to get caught at the starting line when we feel we have to compete with over 40's sex symbols like Joan Collins who was born beautiful, or Jane Fonda who has Henry to thank for her genes. But, we do have it within us to regenerate our own best selves. And, we can do this at any age. The problem is that we get stuck with the idea of chronological age, when it's biological age that counts.

At 50 you can have the body of a 30-year-old or a 70-year-old. It depends on the care you put into it. (After all, 50 percent of aging relates to sedentary living.) Of course, it would have been better if you had started a good and consistent diet and exercise regime at 20. But even now, by following the principles set forth in the upcoming chapters, you can reverse the aging process.

The only thing that keeps you from achieving health, fitness, and good looks at your age is attitude. You have to give up the *give up* attitude, the one that says "my youth is gone, so what?" You can't look like you did at 20, and any attempt to do so is a mistake. You don't want to look "cute" or "perky." Did you ever see anyone looking "cute" at mid-life, frills, flips, and rosebud cheeks? It's a depressing sight that gives middle age a bad name.

What you want to be is a tony, gorgeous woman of 40 plus. When someone remarks, "You don't look 50," you want to say (as Gloria Steinem did), "This is what 50 looks like."

Think Geraldine Ferraro, not Edith Bunker. Forget "fussy"; forget, "flab," "spread," "dowdy," "matronly," and "over-the-hill." Forget all the words you've ever heard coined for middle age. Dare to look and feel better than you ever did.

You *can* do it. Flab *can* be reversed. You *can* be thinner and more flexible. You *can* run a mile, five miles, ten, restore your energy, glow with health, get rid of the feeling that there is no more life to be lived.

Dare to let your hair go gray. Or highlight it with a glimmer of golden brown. Put on a bright red lipstick. Make your eyes look brighter and wider with pink eye shadow. Throw out your dowdy old clothes; start anew.

Startle your husband. Wear azure blue, or watermelon, or taxi-cab yellow. Stand taller, but don't wear high-heeled shoes if they make your feet and legs ache. Wear sexy black patent leather flats and great silky stockings. Buy a new fragrance. Put a fragrant oil lamp near your bed and make lots of love.

Be outrageous, dance, be silly, laugh, increase your laugh lines. Angels fly because they take themselves lightly.

It annoyed me when I was young and serious that my Aunt Myrtle would never tell anyone her age. I know now she did it less for vanity than a desire not to be placed in a certain slot in time. *She* danced, still does. She is, I recently found out, 87. When Claudette Colbert, now 82 plus, was asked how she had so much stamina, she replied, "I just think of myself as 60 with 20 years to go."

Attitude is everything. Instead of slipping into your husband's old Lacostes like I did, or into a middle-aged spread like Betty, work on yourself. Enhance; redo, if necessary. You probably won't end up looking like Linda Evans. That's the roll of the dice. But, you'll be the best version of yourself.

You have to work at it. You can't take your face and body for granted like you once did. You have to be vigilant about diet and exercise, about haircuts, and about putting on sunscreen in the midday sun. You can't think of those things as extras, to do when you have time, like taking in a movie. A beauty and fitness regime must become an integral part of your life.

Health is the cornerstone of beauty at any age, but especially over 40. Without it, you can't possibly look good. No face-lift, tummy tuck, skillfully applied makeup, or $50 haircut will ever replace an agile body, vital skin and hair, and vibrant eyes.

Beauty, as my grandma used to say, comes from within. And that's where we start, with a diet constructed especially for a woman at 40 plus. (You no longer need to be frustrated with diets designed for people your daughter's age.) Our diet not only guarantees weight loss (if *you* stick with it) but also will increase your energy level, your feeling of well-being, and your chance for a long and healthy life. Certain safeguards have been built into this special diet: the required calcium to fight osteoporosis, vitamin E and the B vitamins to combat menopausal stress, and the food guidelines to help prevent heart disease and cancer.

The section on anti-aging exercises will teach you the correct aerobics for your age and body type and how to do them without injuring yourself. It will show you flab-reducing exercises that won't throw your back into traction and stretching exercises that will increase your flexibility and reduce the aches and pains that come from rigid musculature. New visualization and ideokinesiology techniques will realign your body, making you look taller, thinner, and feeling better. And with special breathing exercises you'll learn to restore energy and feel more tranquil.

We'll come out in praise of character lines. ("They're not wrinkles," says skin specialist Lia Schorr. With the aid of Lia Schorr and other experts, you'll learn how to minimize your wrinkles while using your character lines to bring out your own special good looks.

You'll discover how to make gray beautiful and learn when you should give up on it and color your hair. We'll give you flattering hairstyles to choose from, help resolve the long hair-short hair controversy, and teach you everything there is to know about having thicker, glossier hair.

Finish this book and once and for all you'll have a knowledge of the right colors to wear and a great "finally grown-up," sophisticated wardrobe that will cover some of your hard-to-solve figure flaws.

Because it's easy to get down on yourself, we have a whole section called "Sex, Sleep, Scent & Other Rejuvenators," which will make you feel better. It covers everything from music to laughter, sexual fantasies, bubble baths, and meditation. And, all along the way, we will spur you on with real-life stories of women who have taken up the challenge of themselves—women like Lynn Sherman who began running (well, barely) at 41 and who at 49 ran her first New York Marathon.

In the chapter on "Menopause: Myths & Realities," women like yourself will share their experiences, as we work toward bringing the information on this stage of life out of the dark ages. Included will be the latest on osteoporosis and the pros and cons of estrogen replacement therapy.

Near the end of the book, you'll find a chapter on "Flexing Your Mental Muscle." Featured will be a list of resources for the 40-plus woman, like Outward Bound (the adult version), workshops, and fitness camps.

What we do not do is endorse the youth culture. We won't suggest you "cut and stitch" your way back in time. We won't coo at you. We won't make promises we can't keep. (Although we'll ask you to keep a few.) We'll try to fit this beauty and fitness program into your time frame. We won't be phony. We'll try to give you everything you need to know to look fit and fabulous at 40 plus. The rest is up to you.

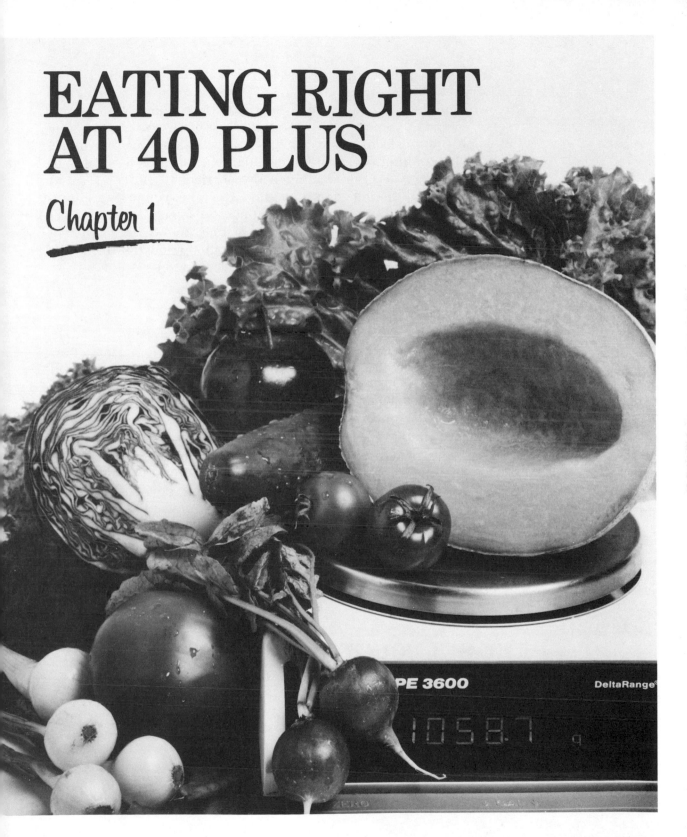

EATING RIGHT
AT 40 PLUS

Chapter 1

I celebrated my 40th birthday by throwing out my collection of neatly typed, alphabetized, color-coded diets that I used to keep in a three-ring binder and read every week or so with the gusto some people reserve for trashy romance novels. I had everything, from the abalone diet (high protein from lots of shellfish; it was tasty but expensive) through the Zen diet (weight loss and higher consciousness through much privation and almost as much brown rice, of course). My diet manifesto had all the ingredients to make it a book-you-just-can't-put-down—relief from a humdrum meat-and-potatoes existence; visions of a svelte, sexy new me through a lunch of macaroons and dinner of martinis (my favorite M diet); and even a dramatic plot about the heroic grapefruit that would destroy all my fat cells in a week.

CRASH DIETS DON'T WORK

My friend Jeanne and I used to spend hours discussing our latest diets. Finding a new diet was like falling in love, but when the love affair ended and we were left pale and irritable and only two pounds lighter at the most, we would be seized with the kind of disillusionment that only a marshmallow hot-fudge banana split can cure. Then we'd make the trek to the ice cream parlor together and order two.

But you should see the two of us now. We're both over 40 and feel and look better than ever—trimmer and more energetic. We've both discovered the real meaning of diet; it's a complete way of life, not a one-week stand with artificial sweeteners. We've recognized that the word diet comes from a Greek word that means "way of life," and we've taken it to heart.

Imagine how I felt when I found out that all those years I'd spent practically starving myself might actually have *kept me from losing weight.* If you need any further inspiration at all to give up crash dieting, consider the Set Point Theory, which holds that a life of calorie cutting can actually make you fat.

THE SET POINT THEORY

Studies show that over half the U.S. population over 30 is overweight or obese, even though the nation has become so calorie-conscious that we've actually eaten less since 1960. Some nutritional experts believe that every time you go on a crash diet and eat less, your body lowers its metabolic rate to compensate for the lower calorie intake. So you need fewer and fewer calories for energy. Hence fewer calories will now make you fat. So it's not far from the truth that a nibble of chocolate could make you gain a pound or two.

We're used to thinking that when you cut calories, your body starts feeding on its own stores of fat. It's true that your body's first reaction is to draw on the most available form of energy when it perceives an emergency, such as less food to burn. But that energy isn't fat, it's glycogen, a form of glucose that's stored in the muscles and the liver. Because glucose is a carbohydrate, you lose it faster than fat. If your crash diet starts out with great results in the first few days, it's because your body has burned glycogen and lost water, which are stored together. But after those few days, the honeymoon with your new diet is over, because now your body will start shedding the tissue it needs the least at the moment. That means if you are used to a sedentary life (if you don't exercise or do physical work), you will lose muscle tissue. If you're overweight and inactive, your body will hang onto its fat because it's a creature of habit, and fat is what it's used to having around.

Worst of all, now that your calorie intake has dropped severely and suddenly, you may laze around even more than usual because your

Diet at Mid-Life: The Myths and Facts

Myth: Your metabolism automatically becomes slower as you age.
Fact: Studies have found that if you let your age slow you down, your body will follow. People who become less active as they get older gain weight, but those who remain physically active and do not gain weight experience little change in metabolic rate.

Myth: As you grow older, the percentage of fat in your body weight increases while your muscle mass decreases.
Fact: This is true only *if* you become sedentary. Those who remain active lose some muscle, but at a much lower rate.

Myth: It becomes harder to digest, absorb, and use the nutrients in the food you eat as you get older.
Fact: Studies do not bear this out. What does increase with age is the use of medications that interfere with normal diges-

tion, absorption, and the utilization of nutrients. Some antacids, for example, interfere with the absorption of several nutrients, and steroids make you excrete more calcium in the urine. Preventive health care will minimize your need for medications so that you won't get caught up in this vicious cycle.

Myth: As you get older, your taste buds lose sensitivity.
Fact: Your taste buds lose sensitivity when you smoke, take certain medicines, or become ill. There's no proof that the ability to taste declines with age.

Myth: Regular bowel movements become more difficult as you get older.
Fact: Unless you have an intestinal disorder, you can guard against constipation at any age by drinking plenty of fluids and including plenty of fiber in your diet, plus exercising regularly.

body is trying to make do with its limited food supply. So you lose energy and enthusiasm and spend more time sleeping. Your fatigue—especially combined with your lack of results—might make you depressed, and there's nothing that makes you gain weight faster than depression because it makes your body even more passive. (Depression also puts you in danger of a chocolate chip binge.)

But you can stop this vicious cycle. *Change your eating habits and start exercising!* Exercise does much more than burn off calories. Thirty minutes of exercise will elevate your metabolic rate for two to four hours after you have finished exercising. This aftereffect can, *without any calorie reduction,* result in an additional weight loss of *four to five pounds a year* if you exercise moderately for 30 minutes a day.

If you're burned out, as I was, by all the low-calorie (low-on-nutrition) diets that do nothing but make you hungry, you will find it difficult to believe (I did) that there is a diet to end all diets, and that it's made up, as it should be, of a sound balance of *all* the nutrients we need at this age to maintain an active and energetic life.

Dr. Audrey Cross, who is a nutritionist at Columbia University and who has countless satisfied slim and healthy clients, composed the Turn-Back-the-Clock Diet (which starts on page 19) especially for this

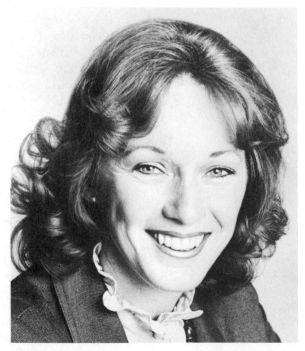

Dr. Audrey Cross

book. In this three-week meal plan (set up to get you started on your own pattern of healthy, low-calorie eating), Dr. Cross has included, for every day, an imaginative range of foods that will spur you on, rather than turn you off, to sticking with your diet.

"If you stick to a wholesome diet, you won't have yearnings for more food," she says. But that's not all that a truly good diet will do for you. It can also help ward off illness, bad moods, and aging.

Even more important to me than the weight I've lost, this way of eating gives me more energy than I've ever experienced (well, since I was about 12).

I find that with this diet and my daily workout, my body feels like a fine-tuned motor, and I don't want to ruin that feeling by pouring down sugar or chemically loaded soft drinks and junk food. The Turn-Back-the-Clock Diet works *best* with daily exercise. The meal plans take into account the active woman's need for extra riboflavin, potassium, iron, zinc, and other nutrients. In a very short time you'll find that exercise, combined with a nutritious and balanced diet, not only creates lean muscle tissue but also wards off depression and sluggishness, making you feel younger. Once you get going with a good diet and exercise plan, you'll wonder why you ever thought it was too late to start!

FINDING YOUR PERFECT WEIGHT

The Lucky Strike cigarette ads of the 1930s, which used to tell figure-conscious young women to "Reach for a Lucky instead of a sweet," belong to the dark ages of health awareness, before anyone actually knew how devastating cigarettes were to the human body. In our era we've had to endure an equally damaging media slogan. Do you recognize this one: "A woman can't be too rich or too thin"? Well, I'm hopeful that in another 10 or 20 years, the anorexic look will be just as passé as smoking. Perhaps as the bulk of the population gets older, we'll also shed the svelte, bikini-clad, 20-year-old figure as the beauty standard against which all women's bodies are measured. I know many beautiful women who are 40 plus, but mature beauty comes from an inner wisdom, from good health, and from staying physically and intellectually active, not from some masochistic attempt to fit into your teenage daughter's designer jeans.

True, if you're overweight, you become a greater health risk as you get older, and your susceptibility to breast cancer and heart disease increases. But now we're starting to find that being too thin can be unhealthy also. When the Metropolitan Life Insurance Company released new weight tables in 1983, based on longevity studies of millions of policyholders who were insured by many different companies, it showed that the ideal weights for longer lives were up to 10 percent higher than the "ideal" weights of 25 years ago.

There is some controversy over the new Metropolitan Life Insurance Company tables—mostly from the American Heart Association. The concern is that these tables will encourage serious problems with overweight that could be damaging to the heart. But it seems fairly certain that your ideal weight at 45 isn't the same as it was when you were 20. Dr. Reubin Andres, who is clinical director of the Gerontology Research Center at the National Institute on Aging, says that the new Metropolitan tables are just about right for people over 40. He believes that height, weight, sex, and age are the criteria for establishing your perfect weight, and your weight should go up some with age. However, before determining the best weight for *you,* you should check with your physician.

You can find your new ideal weight in the Metropolitan Life Insurance Company table shown below. If you're not sure of your frame size, you can find it by measuring your elbow breadth (see instructions and illustration on opposite page).

Metropolitan Life Insurance Company's 1983 Height/Weight Table for Women

Height	Small Frame	Medium Frame	Large Frame
4 ft. 10 in.	102-111	109-121	118-131
4 ft. 11 in.	103-113	111-123	120-134
5 ft. 0 in.	104-115	113-126	122-137
5 ft. 1 in.	106-118	115-129	125-140
5 ft. 2 in.	108-121	118-132	128-143
5 ft. 3 in.	111-124	121-135	131-147
5 ft. 4 in.	114-127	124-138	134-151
5 ft. 5 in.	117-130	127-141	137-155
5 ft. 6 in.	120-133	130-144	140-159
5 ft. 7 in.	123-136	133-147	143-163
5 ft. 8 in.	126-139	136-150	146-167
5 ft. 9 in.	129-142	139-153	149-170
5 ft. 10 in.	132-145	142-156	152-173
5 ft. 11 in.	135-148	145-159	155-176
6 ft. 0 in.	138-151	148-162	158-179

NOTE: Weights are for women aged 25 to 59 and are based on the lowest mortality in this age category. Weight is in pounds according to frame (in indoor clothing weighing 3 pounds and in shoes with 1-in. heels).

HOW TO DETERMINE
YOUR BODY FRAME BY ELBOW BREADTH

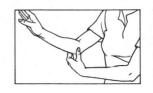

To make a simple approximation of your frame size, extend your arm and bend the forearm upward at a 20-degree angle. Keep the fingers straight and turn the inside of your wrist away from the body. Place the thumb and index finger of your other hand on the two prominent bones on *either side* of your elbow. Measure the distance between your finger and thumb against a ruler or a tape measure. Compare the measurements on the following table.

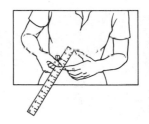

This table lists the elbow measurements for medium-framed women of various heights. Measurements lower than those listed indicate you have a small frame, and higher measurements indicate a large frame.

Height in 1-In. Heels	Elbow Breadth
4 ft. 10 in.-4 ft. 11 in.	2¼ in.-2½ in.
5 ft. 0 in.-5 ft. 3 in.	2¼ in.-2½ in.
5 ft. 4 in.-5 ft. 7 in.	2⅜ in.-2⅝ in.
5 ft. 8 in.-5 ft. 11 in.	2⅜ in.-2⅝ in.
6 ft. 0 in.	2½ in.-2¾ in.

THE McAERDLE FORMULA
(HOW MUCH FAT IS REALLY ON YOUR BODY?)

If your weight is a few pounds under or over what the weight table says it should be, don't panic; you're most likely still within the normal weight range. Though having some body fat is important, having too much or too little means it's time to adjust your eating and exercise habits.

To find out how much body fat you have, follow these four simple steps and circle the appropriate measurement numbers on the accompanying table.

1. Measure your waist, placing the tape measure ½ inch above your navel.

2. Measure your right thigh, placing the tape measure just below your buttocks.

3. Measure your right forearm at the widest part between your elbow and your wrist.

4. Next to your measurements on the table is a constant number. Circle this number, and use it to fill in the formula at the bottom of the table. Add and subtract the numbers where indicated. Your final number will tell you what percentage of fat your body is.

Waist		Right Thigh		Right Forearm	
Measurement (in.)	Constant	Measurement (in.)	Constant	Measurement (in.)	Constant
20	27	14	29	6	26
21	28	15	31	7	30
22	29	16	33	8	34
23	31	17	35	9	39
24	32	18	37	10	43
25	33	19	40	11	47
26	35	20	42	12	52
27	36	21	44	13	56
28	37	22	46	14	60
29	39	23	48	15	65
30	40	24	50	16	69
31	41	25	52	17	73
32	43	26	54	18	78
33	44	27	56	19	82
34	45	28	58	20	86
35	47	29	60		
36	48	30	62		
37	49	31	65		
38	51	32	67		
39	52	33	69		
40	53	34	71		

WAIST CONSTANT NUMBER _____

PLUS (+) _____

THIGH CONSTANT NUMBER _____

SUBTOTAL _____

MINUS (−) _____

FOREARM CONSTANT NUMBER _____

SUBTOTAL _____

MINUS 20 (− 20) _____

APPROXIMATE BODY FAT
   PERCENTAGE _____ %

If the percentage of your body fat is 30 or more, you need to lose some weight and increase or begin exercising. If your percentage is less than 17, you should be eating more. If your percentage is 18 to 29, your body fat is within normal range; you don't have to worry about your weight.

WE ARE WHAT WE EAT

I'm not saying that you shouldn't lose weight, because a balanced diet of controlled proportions, combined with exercise, will help you reach, and keep, your ideal weight. I am saying that we can all throw off our dieting chains. We can look and feel better than ever with a healthy diet. Our clothes will fit better, and people around us will notice the terrific, glowing look of well-being. But the rewards of good nutrition go far beyond just the way you look. You will also feel better, not only because you'll be healthier and more trim but because you'll be able to fight the aging effects of stress and the "blues." Diet, you see, can have a profound effect upon your moods.

MOOD FOOD

Psychologist Arthur C. Hochberg is continually appalled at the number of patients he sees who are taking prescription Valium to help them cope with major ordeals in life, such as a divorce, a death in the family, or career crises. Hochberg finds that many of the doctors who give patients tranquilizing drugs never even ask about their intake of alcohol, nicotine, caffeine, or sugar. He feels that people who pacify themselves with cocktails or candy are probably creating a nutritional deficiency that puts their bodies under even more stress. Stress wears down the body's immunity. Hochberg, in fact, believes that most illnesses are the result of an exaggerated or prolonged reaction to stress.

So what do you do when you're under stress? Start forming healthier habits, and try using food properly to reduce tension. Hochberg recommends a program of reduced animal protein, with increased complex carbohydrates (that means lots of whole grains, vegetables, and fruit). For the nervous munchies, he suggests snacks of raw almonds; sunflower seeds; nonprocessed cheeses; unsalted, unbuttered popcorn; and yogurt. (Flavor yogurt with your own fresh fruit and avoid the six extra teaspoons of sugar that commercial flavored yogurt typically has.) Munch on these foods as often as you like, but keep to small quantities whenever you do. By eating this way, you're continuously feeding your body with high-grade complex carbohydrates that balance your blood sugar levels and nourish your adrenal glands, which become exhausted under tension.

It may be hard to withdraw from caffeine if you have a habit of drinking coffee to wipe out that fatigue brought on by stress. But the last thing your body really needs is more stress-inducing caffeine. I used to be a coffee addict, but when it began to take its toll on my nervous stomach, I knew I had to stop. I managed to withdraw cold turkey by drinking decaffeinated French roast. Keep plenty of herbal caffeine-free teas and coffees on hand at home and at the office. There is an amazing variety with which to indulge yourself.

But maybe you choose to console yourself with cookies when you're under stress. You do that because it actually works—sugars and starches have been found to have a calming effect. That's because carbohydrates raise the level of a brain chemical called serotonin that is associated with feeling relaxed, calm, sleepy, less depressed, and less sensitive to pain.

Newborn babies fall asleep faster when L-tryptophan, the amino acid that also triggers the serotonin levels in the brain, and carbohydrates are added to their formulas. This combination can work for adults, too. This doesn't mean you should put down this book and head for the nearest bakery. But you should ensure that your diet has a variety of complex carbohydrates that give you a constant sense of well-being.

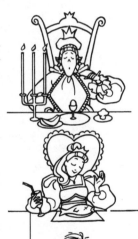

Eat Several Small Meals a Day
and All before 8:00 P.M.

In a study conducted by Dr. Walter Mertz, a nutritionist with the U.S. Department of Agriculture's Caloric Research Laboratory, it was found that people who ate their calories (1,200 of them) over several meals a day lost more weight than those who ate them (also 1,200 calories) all in one meal.

Dr. Mertz also found that those who ate most of their 1,200 calories at breakfast and lunch lost more weight than those who ate most of their 1,200 calories at dinner.

The moral: Eat like a queen at breakfast, a princess at lunch, and a pauper at dinner. Eat your last meal before 8:00 P.M. so you have time to burn off calories. And nosh on low-calorie snacks, such as fruit and raw veggies in between meals.

Know that L-tryptophan isn't a quick shot that relaxes you—L-trypto-phan-rich foods such as turkey, tuna, dairy products, and peanuts should be part of your daily diet, so that you feel more relaxed all the time and more able to cope with stress.

However, if you want to be alert in the afternoon, you might try having your main protein meal for lunch. A recent study at Harvard found that people over 40 feel more alert if they have high-protein lunches. But don't make it a banquet. Your thinking becomes less sharp after a heavy 1,000-calorie lunch than after a small one. Grazing—eating as many as six small meals a day instead of three large ones—is very much in vogue right now, and if you stick to healthy grazing food (fruits or raw vegetables midmorning and midafternoon), this practice can keep your blood sugar level, and hence your moods, on an even keel.

To relax in the evening, and later sleep well, try a high complex-carbohydrate meal for dinner—pasta or rice with vegetables.

Another word to the wise—if you want to feel up and positive, don't drink. Alcohol has a negative effect on moods. A study at the University of California found that women who drink even moderately (more than two drinks twice a week) experience increased depression, anger, and mental confusion—and sobering up doesn't help the bad mood. Cut back to two drinks a week, or less, and see if you feel happier. Alcohol is full of calories, anyway, and nothing makes you feel quite as terrible as waking up with a hangover. Lately, I've found that mineral water, salt-free seltzer with a twist of lemon or lime, or a light alcoholic beverage, like a wine spritzer—half wine, half seltzer—is all I need as a before-dinner drink or something to sip through an entire evening.

MEMORY FOOD

Studies have shown that alcohol may interfere with memory as you get older. They have also shown that certain foods may help improve your memory. Acetylcholine is the substance in the brain that helps us remember things. Older people generally have lower levels of acetylcho-line than younger people because, when you get older, your body may break down this substance more rapidly. But you may be able to build up your body's supply of acetylcholine by starting right now to eat a diet rich in lecithin, or choline, which the body converts to acetylcho-line. Eggs, dairy products, wheat germ, and soybeans are excellent sources of lecithin, and you can also buy powdered lecithin in a natural foods store. It's unflavored, so you can mix it with water, soups, or juices. A good step—just don't expect to suddenly have the memory of an elephant.

FIGHTING OSTEOPOROSIS

Did you know that one-third of all the women in the United States get fewer vitamins, minerals, and other nutrients than they need? We've all heard about our Western diseases of excess, such as cardiovascular disease, high blood pressure, and many forms of cancer. But modern science is now beginning to discover the ways that we're malnourished. Eating too little of the right kinds of food can put us at higher risk for the problems we have to guard against as we get older. Studies of high blood pressure patients, for instance, have revealed that the disease seems to go hand in hand with a deficiency of calcium.

The diet we give you at the end of this chapter has twice the current Recommended Dietary Allowance of calcium, which is 800 milligrams, because this is one mineral that women need more and more of the older they get. If you weren't calcium-conscious enough to make it an important part of your diet (in either foods or supplements) when you were younger, you should start now, as a weapon against osteoporosis.

Our bodies stop building and strengthening bones at about 35, so you're already losing calcium from your bones. But the rate of bone loss becomes even more rapid during menopause because your body begins to lose estrogen, which helps to protect the calcium supply. (See chapter 8 for more information.) If you don't give your body the calcium it needs, as you get older your bones could become very brittle and easily break.

Up to 40 percent of American women may eventually develop osteoporosis. Here is a list of factors, reprinted from *The Calcium Bible* by Patricia Hausman, M.S. (New York: Rawson Associates, 1985), that increase your risk. How many of these apply to you?

✓ a low-calcium intake

✓ a thin or petite frame

✓ a sedentary life-style

✓ a high-stress life-style

✓ a family history of loss of height or hip fracture in later life

✓ removal of the ovaries

✓ absence of any pregnancies

✓ the smoking habit

✓ overconsumption of alcohol

✓ long-term use of drugs interfering with calcium metabolism

✓ Caucasian race

✓ an ethnic background of British, northern European, Chinese, or Japanese extraction

If you are at risk, and even if you aren't—protect yourself by taking a calcium carbonate or calcium lactate supplement. A warning: Avoid dolomite or supplements made from bone meal as both substances

How Common Is Osteoporosis?

Osteoporosis has become so common that most experts call it an epidemic. Up to 40 percent of American women may eventually develop it. Here are some facts to help you size up the problem:[1]

✔ Every year more than half a million American women join the ranks of those afflicted with osteoporosis.

✔ Statisticians record more than two million bone fractures a year among American women aged 45 or older. Osteoporosis accounts for at least three-fourths of the fractures.

✔ About 40,000 American women die each year from complications of osteoporosis. The immobility that a broken bone may cause increases the risk of infections such as pneumonia, blood clots, and embolisms in the lungs that cut off the vital supply of blood.

1. Reprinted with permission of Rawson Associates, from *The Calcium Bible*, by Patricia Hausman, M.S. Copyright 1985 by Patricia Hausman.

(still plentiful on the shelves of natural foods stores) sometimes have a high lead content. You should also consume the following calcium-laden foods: sardines; salmon; herring; mackerel; low-fat cheese, milk, and yogurt; tofu; and green, leafy vegetables (the darker the lettuce, the more calcium in it).

FIGHTING FATTY FOODS

An unhealthy diet makes it difficult for you to absorb calcium. Too much fat can bind up the calcium in a form that's useless to your body. Alcohol, especially more than two drinks a day, can also make it difficult for your body to absorb calcium. And too much protein will cause your body to excrete calcium in urine, so try cutting back on meat. A delicious, calcium-rich main dish is a stir fry with half a serving of beef or chicken, substituting tofu (soy protein cheese) cubes for the other half.

There are many other reasons, of course, to purge fats (especially the saturated animal fats) from your diet, starting with atherosclerosis, the abnormal thickening and hardening of the artery walls. Your heart, like every other muscle, needs a good supply of blood from your arteries.

Dietary Guidelines for Americans

Here are the latest nutrition guidelines, compiled by the U.S. Department of Agriculture.[2]

✔ Eat a variety of foods daily in adequate amounts, including selections of: fruits; vegetables; whole grain and enriched breads, cereals, and other products made from grains; milk, cheese, yogurt, and other products made from milk; meats; poultry; fish; eggs; and dried beans and peas.

✔ Maintain desirable weight by eating slowly, taking smaller portions and avoiding seconds, eating a variety of foods low in calories and high in nutrients, and increasing physical activity.

✔ Avoid too much fat, saturated fat, and cholesterol by means of the following: choose lean meats, fish, poultry, and dried beans as protein sources; use egg yolks and organ meats moderately; limit your intake of butter, cream, lard, heavily hydrogenated fats (some margarines), shortenings, and foods containing palm and coconut oils; trim fat off meats; broil, bake, or boil rather than fry; moderate your use of foods that contain fat, such as breaded and deep-fried foods; read labels carefully to determine both amount and type of fat present in foods.

✔ Eat more foods with adequate starch and fiber: whole grain breads and cereals, fruits, vegetables, and dried beans and peas; and more starchy foods in place of those that have large amounts of fats and sugars.

✔ Avoid excessive sugar by using less of sugars and foods containing large amounts of sugars including white sugar, brown sugar, raw sugar, honey, and syrups (soft drinks, candies, cakes, and cookies); avoid sweets between meals; read labels for clues on sugar content (if the name sugar, sucrose, glucose, maltose, dextrose, lactose, fructose, or syrup appears first, there is a large amount of sugar); select fresh fruits or fruits processed without syrup, or with light, rather than heavy, syrup.

✔ Avoid too much sodium by learning to enjoy the flavors of unsalted foods; cooking without salt or with only small amounts of added salt; flavoring foods with lemon juice; adding little or no salt to food at the table; limiting your intake of salty foods such as potato chips and pretzels, pickled foods, cured meats, some cheese, and some canned foods; checking labels to determine sodium content; using lower sodium products when available to replace the usual choices that have higher sodium content.

✔ If you drink alcoholic beverages at all, do so in moderation.

2. U.S. Department of Agriculture in conjunction with the U.S. Department of Human Nutrition Information Services. *Nutrition and Your Health: Dietary Guidelines for Americans,* 2d ed. Washington, D.C., 1985.

When cholesterol and other fatty substances begin clogging the inner walls of the coronary arteries, making them like stopped-up water pipes, you begin to be a prime candidate for heart disease.

Beef, pork, lamb, egg yolks, butter, cream, ice cream, whole milk, and cream cheese are all fatty foods, and we're better off limiting our intake of them as we get older. If you eat meat, make sure it's a lean cut, with all visible fat trimmed off. With dairy foods eat only the skim or low-fat variety. The solid and hydrogenated vegetable shortenings, coconut oil, and palm oil, which are often used in commercial baked goods and nondairy milk and cream substitutes, are also enemies of good health.

But don't think for a moment that the body doesn't need some fat. Fats carry the fat-soluble vitamins A, D, E, and K. They can even help keep us looking youthful because they aid in keeping our skin from drying out. Fish oils and vegetable oils—sunflower, safflower, corn, soybean and so forth—are fine since they don't turn into artery sludge as readily as animal fats do. In fact, scientists say fish oils and vegetable oils may actually help your heart and arteries resist disease.

Instead of eating bad fats in your diet, eat more fiber—fresh, whole fruits and vegetables and whole grain breads and cereals. Avocados and coconuts are the only fruits that are high in fats and should be only a small part of your diet. But a little avocado spread on a sandwich is OK as a delicious substitute for butter or mayonnaise. Avocado is an excellent source of potassium, too.

You need dairy products for calcium, but stick to the skim or low-fat kinds. I thought I couldn't live without butter on my baked potato until I tried using low-fat ricotta cheese, low-fat cottage cheese, or yogurt on it.

I've also made poultry (removing the fatty skin before cooking) a major part of my diet, since I've gotten away from eating red meats. If you *must* eat red meats and pork (which have been allowed in *our* diet at the end of the chapter), eat only the lean cuts. Many livestock breeders as well as the manufacturers of meat products are now aware of the public's health consciousness and are reducing the amount of fat in their products. The packaging, however, must say lean beef, pork, or lamb, or don't buy it.

Your goal should be to decrease the amount of fat in your diet by 8 to 10 percent of your calorie intake. (The fat in the typical American diet is 40 percent of calories.)

SAY NO TO SALT

The other enemy of a healthy heart is salt. Excessive salt consumption can cause a buildup of body fluids in your system, making it difficult for your heart to pump blood through the cardiovascular system. This can result in high blood pressure, which might cause a heart attack or stroke. Beware of processed and canned foods. Many canned soups and vegetables are heavily salted. If you do buy canned foods, choose "low salt" or low-sodium varieties now offered by some manufacturers who are sensitive to the problem.

If you must resort to using canned vegetables, rinse the salt away in clear water. You won't miss salt if you start cooking with herbs and spices. Keep pepper, thyme, oregano, basil, curry, cinnamon, chili, tarragon, onion and garlic powders, fresh onions, garlic, green pepper, lemon juice, and flavored vinegar on hand. Let your imagination run wild when you're cooking. If you use fresh herbs and spices, you'll get an extra bonus on flavor and nutrients.

My favorite salt-free snack, by the way, is hot-air-popped popcorn. Without salt or oil, it offers multi-nutrients for a minimum of calories. Sometimes I season it with some chopped fresh herbs, grated low-fat cheese, or a little garlic powder. I even take my own bag to the movies. I figure that those who stand in line to buy the overpriced, oiled and salted variety don't know what I know!

FOOD AND CANCER

Selenium is a controversial mineral that might eventually prove to be essential in warding off cancer. In any number of animal experiments since 1949, it has reduced the incidence of colon, breast, liver, and other body tumors, and it's possible that a small daily dose in supplements (not more than 100 micrograms since more could be toxic) will someday be part of our daily vitamin supplements. Selenium comes from the soil, and if you live in South Dakota, Wyoming, New Mexico, or Utah, there is so much of it in your soil that you can be reassured that your home-grown grains, vegetables, and meat supply all the selenium you need. But wherever you live, there are a number of foods that are especially good sources of selenium—whole wheat bread, cereals, and pasta; mushrooms; asparagus; meats (especially organ meats); and dairy products.

The American Cancer Society has yet to take a position on selenium, but the society's seven guidelines for avoiding cancer should be engraved on every refrigerator. So far, no one has devised a complete

The American Cancer Society's Seven Diet Guidelines

Although there is no actual anti-cancer diet, many scientists now feel that what we eat and *don't* eat can lower our risk of getting the disease. Ernst L. Wynder, M.D., president of the American Health Foundation in New York City, believes that up to one-half of all cancers in women are related to diet.

The American Cancer Society has made the following suggestions that many cancer experts feel are worth following:

1. Avoid obesity.

2. Reduce the saturated and unsaturated fat in your diet by 10 percent. Cut down on your daily intake of fatty meats, whole-milk dairy products, butter, cooking oils, and fats.

3. Increase your fiber intake (by double or about 30 grams a day).

4. Eat foods rich in vitamins C and A (with beta-carotene).

5. Eat vegetables from the mustard family (cruciferous family) such as broccoli, cabbage, cauliflower, and brussels sprouts.

6. Avoid salt-cured, smoked, or nitrate-processed meat (such as hot dogs).

7. If you drink, be moderate.

anti-cancer diet, but we know that vitamins A and C, as well as cabbage and other vegetables from the mustard family, seem to retard or prevent the growth of cancer, while fats and nitrates enhance it. Ernst L. Wynder, M.D., president of the American Health Foundation, believes that up to one-half of all cancers in women—and one-third in men—are related to nutrition. Knowing this I think it would be folly not to improve your diet.

The risk of cancer—particularly breast cancer, at this stage of our lives—is why many women should start eating right and getting in shape, even if it's for the first time, when they hit the ripe side of 40. As I mentioned earlier, I'll gladly step into any crusade against the starveling look, but at the same time, I can't stress enough how bad obesity is for your health. If you're concerned about breast cancer—and who isn't—there's strong evidence that being overweight, especially in the postmenopausal years, brings on higher levels of your own estrogen, which seem to increase breast cancer risk.

Being fat and *eating* fat put women at risk for breast cancer. It appears that saturated fat is in league with estrogen. Women who eat meat, and hence a lot of animal fat, have been found to process estrogen differently from vegetarian women, who eat about one-third the fat that omnivores do. The meat eaters recycle more estrogen in their blood, while the vegetarians pass more out of the body. And vegetarians also seem to have higher levels of DHEA, the cancer protective hormone.

NIX SUGAR AND ITS SUBSTITUTES

I've just about given up sugar, honey, molasses, and any chemical substitute and now use sweet, natural fruit juices in cooking instead of sugar most of the time. You just can't win with sugar and its substitutes; they just provide (or encourage you to consume) empty calories that don't really satisfy your appetite.

DRINK THE BEST

Say good-bye to diet soft drinks. Say hello to water instead. You should drink six to eight glasses of some healthy liquid a day (it could be soup), and at least two or three of these should be water. At mealtime, water helps you swallow and digest food. Water also helps the kidneys function and never interferes with the absorption of nutrients. Water with a bit of lemon juice is a safe, gentle laxative.

I can offer no such words of praise for sodas that have off-tasting sugar substitutes, or for those loaded with sugar and caffeine. I've already mentioned that I've switched to noncaffeinated coffees, something I thought I'd never be able to do, but found to be not so tough at all. I did it because my gynecologist Dr. Niels Lauersen told me that his patients notice a reduction in benign breast lumps within two years after they stop consuming caffeinated products, such as coffee, tea, cola, and chocolate.

DIET IS A MAJOR HEALTH FACTOR

By now it must seem that diet is everything. Well, it does have an astounding effect on our health. In the mid-1970s, J. A. Scharffenberg, M.D., at the San Joaquin Community Hospital, Bakersfield, California, conducted a study that was called the Health Consequences of a Good Life-style. He concluded that to have a long and healthy life, you need a good diet (which includes eating breakfast), adequate exercise appropriate for your age and body-frame weight, enough sleep, little or no alcohol, no smoking, and, of course, happiness. If you keep up all these good health habits, you can add about nine years to your life, or put your life expectancy at around 85. Good health habits not only could increase your life expectancy but give you the vim, vigor, and vitality of someone 30 years younger.

IT ALL STARTS AT THE SUPERMARKET

You might keep Dr. Scharffenberg's study in mind whenever you go to the supermarket. It's easy to make a resolution to stick to a healthy diet, but it is hard to keep it with cookies, fatty cheeses, soda, ice cream, pastries, and all those "easy-on-your-time, but hard-on-your-health" convenience foods staring you in the face. In one survey, 78 percent of the shoppers who responded said that their snack food purchases were made on impulse.

But that carton of ice cream doesn't jump into your cart as you stroll by. Your children are probably adults or almost adults, so no one will grab the "undesirables" if you don't. Temptation is hard to resist, there's no doubt about that. So arm yourself with these tips: Never shop on an empty stomach; eat a healthy meal before you shop; and write out a shopping list ahead of time and resolve to stick to it. (Marketers *do* respond to shifts in consumer demand, so your choices will help make healthier alternatives more available to all.)

About that shopping list. You may have some items on it that need revising. You're going for a change in your cuisine, so slowly introduce some alternatives to your old standbys. Is rice on your shopping list? Make sure it's enriched or whole grain brown rice. Buy fresh vegetables whenever possible. Reach for low-sodium mineral water or seltzer instead of soda. Buy fruit juice to mix with seltzer to make juice "spritzers." Buy popcorn instead of potato chips, and pop it yourself without salt or butter. Buy more chicken, turkey, and fish and less red meat. Roast a turkey or chicken early in the week, and keep it in the refrigerator for sandwiches, to preempt the salami and liverwurst.

THE TURN-BACK-THE-CLOCK DIET

The Turn-Back-the-Clock Diet was designed by Dr. Audrey Cross, a nutritionist, to help you develop a *permanent* healthy eating style, with a variety of food that tastes wonderful and contains all the nutrients you need. Each day's menu meets the Recommended Dietary Allowances (RDA) for vitamin A, thiamine, riboflavin, niacin, vitamin C, phosphorus, and iron. The calcium levels exceed the current RDA because women our age need more than the population average. The B vitamins and choline in these menus exceed 100 percent of the RDA, as do the beta-carotene and vitamin A sources. We've also included the major sources of selenium each day and kept the cholesterol and sodium at a healthy level. For sodium, that's below 2,000 milligrams a day; for cholesterol, less than 250 milligrams.

This is a diet your entire family can enjoy! You don't have to eat a different menu from the rest of them because there is enough variety, taste, and texture in this diet to keep everyone interested. For family members who aren't worried about calories, meal portions can be larger. And nondieting members can add all the fruits and vegetables that they want to their meal. Because the diet is 25 percent protein, it's best not to increase protein portions, but to add on the complex carbohydrates.

This 1,000-calorie-a-day plan has been set up for one person. But this meal can be doubled, tripled, or quadrupled in order to stretch to all family members. Dr. Cross says that it can be increased in this manner without changing the taste or texture of the meals.

The person who doesn't exercise will lose about two pounds a week on this diet (a reasonable amount of weight to lose in this period of time) if she sticks to the recommended portions. It's also necessary to stay with the correctly alloted portions and to eat everything on the menu in order to get the required nutrients.

For every 30 minutes you exercise each day, you should add an additional 150 to 200 calories taken from fruits and vegetables. (See the calorie tables on pages 36–40.)

Once you have achieved your ideal weight, you can maintain this diet as a lifelong pursuit by substituting certain foods for others. For example, substitute a piece of chicken for a lean piece of roast pork. The point is that you become accustomed to a *new* way of eating—one that is composed of a balanced diet that is heavy on the complex carbohydrates and one that sticks to a certain limited portion of foods.

At first you should weigh or measure your foods (after cooking them) to become accustomed to the amount you should dish up for yourself. Once you've eyed these portions, you will be able to judge for yourself how large or small they should be.

The Turn-Back-the-Clock Diet is full of fresh vegetables, fruits, whole grains, and pasta. You eat much less protein (only 25 percent), less than the traditional American diet calls for, and cut down drastically on cholesterol, sugar, and caffeine.

In this diet are cruciferous vegetables, which are members of the mustard family (see page 22), and those containing beta-carotene. Both types have been recommended by the American Cancer Society because they are richly contained in the diets of societies that have low incidences of cancer. The diet includes plenty of fiber, which has been recommended as a preventive measure against colon cancer and other digestive tract diseases. It also includes substitutes for butter and other high-fat foods that contribute to atherosclerosis, heart disease, and cancer.

THE RULES FOR THE TURN-BACK-THE-CLOCK DIET

✔ Do not eat anything that is battered, fried, sauced, gravied, buttered, or creamed. If you steam vegetables over water instead of boiling them in the liquid, you'll seal in all the natural vitamins, minerals, flavor, and consistency. Meats and fowl that you cook with steam or roast on a rack will have surprisingly fewer calories and less cholesterol because the fat drips down into the liquid below.

✔ Use no butter, margarine, mayonnaise, salad dressing, cream, sour cream, or other fats. (Use a nonstick pan for omelets and the like.)

✔ Use no sugar or artificial sweeteners.

✔ Eat everything on the menu.

✔ Do not eat more than is allowed—measure it.

✔ Prepare unprocessed fresh foods whenever possible.

✔ Use whole fruits rather than juices. If you substitute one fruit for another, make sure it is the required size. For example, if you substitute a banana for a kiwi fruit because you can't find one locally, or for a persimmon because it's out of season, make sure it is one-half of a banana because that is the size this diet requires you to eat.

✔ Eat whole grain breads and cereals (the word wheat alone does not mean whole wheat).

✔ Drink lots of fluids—water, regular, mineral, and sparkling; decaffeinated black coffee; and tea. Don't drink undiluted fruit juices; they have too many calories—too much condensed sugar content, even if it's natural. If you do drink them, cut them in half with water.

✔ Do not use spreads on sandwiches. The lettuce called for will keep them from tasting dry.

✔ Carry sandwiches from home; if ordered at a deli or cafe, be sure to tell the waitress to "hold the mayo!"

✔ For lunch carry salads from home or assemble them at fast-food restaurants.

✔ Always substitute a citrus fruit for another citrus fruit.

✔ Substitute one menu meal for another (dinner for a dinner, etc.), but do not skip a meal.

✔ Eat exactly what is on the menu in the *exact* portions given to get all your necessary nutrients.

✔ Note that a one-inch cube of cheese is equal to one ounce.

✔ To feed a family, double, triple, or quadruple meal menus, as required.

✔ If cooking for one, freeze extra portions to use later.

✔ To maintain your diet, repeat meals from the three-week plan. Also begin to recognize the rhythm of the diet. For breakfast there is usually cereal, skim milk, and a fruit. For lunch you have a salad or sandwich. For dinner a protein, starch, two vegetables, a salad, and fruit.

✔ If you use canned or frozen vegetables or fruits, don't worry that you will be cheated of nutrients. These are usually frozen or packed shortly after they are picked, often making them fresher than "fresh" produce that has traveled a long distance from where it was grown to the supermarket. Ideally, the food you eat should be grown in your own garden.

✔ When eating out, eat one piece of bread with no butter, no more. "Better to eat a breadstick, as it's more satisfying," says Dr.

Cross. Ask that your vegetables be prepared without fats such as butter, margarine, or oil. If they come to you looking shiny (a visible sign of fats), send them back.

✔ If some foods on this diet are not available in your local supermarket, ask for them again and again, and have your friends ask for them too. Consumer pressure works.

Cruciferous Vegetables

Cruciferous vegetables are members of the mustard family. Eating lots of these types of vegetables is recommended by the American Cancer Society.

When selecting these vegetables, look for the freshest, crispest, and most brightly colored leaves with no wilting or yellowing. Look for cauliflower and broccoli whose flowers are tight and unopened and for cabbage that is moist and shiny. Check turnips and kohlrabi for firmness.

When preparing these vegetables, never overcook!

Here is a list of some members included in this family:

Broccoli	Chinese vegetables	Rutabagas
Brussels sprouts	such as bok choy	Mustard greens
Cabbage,	Collard greens	Turnip greens
green and white	Horseradish	Turnips
Cauliflower	Kohlrabi	Watercress
Chinese broccoli	Radishes	
and Chinese		
cabbage		

Menus for 21 Days
The Turn-Back-the-Clock Diet

DAY 1
BREAKFAST
> 1 cup hot oatmeal
> ½ of a small banana
> 1 cup skim milk

LUNCH
> 1 sandwich made with:
>> 2 slices cracked wheat bread, 1 slice Swiss cheese, and 4 leaves Boston lettuce
>
> Green bean salad made with:
>> 1 cup cooked green beans, marinated in 1 tablespoon lemon juice, ¼ teaspoon dillweed, and a dash of black pepper
>
> 1 small peach

DINNER
> 3 ounces fresh shrimp poached in:
>> ¼ cup white wine and a fresh basil leaf
>
> Rice pilaf made with:
>> ½ cup cooked enriched rice, 1 tablespoon chopped onions, ¼ cup bouillon (low-salt), ¼ cup chopped fresh parsley, and ¼ cup frozen peas
>
> ½ cup cooked carrots sprinkled lightly with nutmeg
> Small salad made with:
>> 1 cup romaine lettuce, ¼ cup shredded red cabbage, and 1 teaspoon balsamic or wine vinegar

SNACK
> ½ cup low-fat plain yogurt
> ¼ cup fresh or frozen blueberries

DAY 2
BREAKFAST
> Omelet made with:
>> ¼ cup sliced fresh mushrooms, 1 large egg, and 1 egg white
>
> 1 small cloverleaf roll
> 1 teaspoon sugar-free orange marmalade*
> ¼ cup fresh grapefruit sections

LUNCH
> Salad bar salad made with:
>> 1 cup each of iceberg lettuce and loose-leaf lettuce; and ¼ cup each of beets, wax beans, red kidney beans, shredded red cabbage, chopped celery, and lemon juice
>
> 1 medium Granny Smith apple

DINNER
> 3 ounces fresh pork roast (lean meat only), baked
> ½ medium sweet potato, baked in the skin
> 1 cup cooked mustard greens
> 1 medium corn bread muffin†
> Small salad made with:
>> ½ cup shredded cabbage, 1 tablespoon chopped sweet red peppers, ¼ teaspoon caraway seeds, and 1 tablespoon lemon juice

SNACK
> 1 slice of watermelon

*Sorrell Ridge is a sugar-free marmalade.
†Make your own, eliminating sugar and honey. To give muffin a sweet taste, mix nonfat dry milk with apple juice and use as the liquid in the recipe.

DAY 3

BREAKFAST
2 slices raisin bread, enriched, without sugar
2 teaspoons peanut butter
1 cup skim milk
¼ of a small cantaloupe

LUNCH
Chicken stir fry made with:
3 ounces lean chicken; ¼ cup each of sliced fresh mushrooms and snow peas; 2 tablespoons each of bamboo shoots, chopped onions, and chopped celery
¼ cup cooked enriched rice
2 small plums

DINNER
Italian salad made with:
1 cup Bibb lettuce; ½ cup spinach; ¼ cup each of shredded carrots, chopped cauliflower, and garbanzo beans; 1 can water-packed sardines; 1 ounce Provolone cheese, cubed; 2 teaspoons wine vinegar; and ¼ teaspoon oregano
1 slice enriched Italian bread

SNACK
10 to 12 red grapes

DAY 4

BREAKFAST
1 shredded wheat biscuit, unsweetened
1 cup skim milk
¼ cup fresh or frozen strawberries

LUNCH
1 large tomato, stuffed with:
3 ounces water-packed tuna, served on a bed of lettuce
2 saltine crackers (low-salt)
1 medium Granny Smith apple

DINNER
Italian minestrone made with:
½ cup each of red kidney beans, cubed zucchini, canned tomatoes with liquid, and bouillon (low-salt); 2 tablespoons chopped onions; ¼ cup frozen spinach; and a dash of oregano and garlic powder
1 slice enriched Italian bread
1 ounce low-fat mozzarella cheese
Small salad made with:
1 cup red-leaf lettuce and 1 tablespoon low-calorie Italian dressing

SNACK
1 small Bosc pear, poached in ¼ cup white grape juice

DAY 5

BREAKFAST

    1 cup low-fat plain yogurt

    ½ cup fresh or frozen blueberries

LUNCH

    1 sandwich made with:

        2 slices pumpernickel bread, 1 ounce American or cheddar cheese, 2 lettuce leaves, 3 or 4 thin cucumber slices, 1 or 2 thinly sliced fresh mushrooms

15 to 20 Thompson seedless grapes

DINNER

    5 to 6 ounces roast leg of lamb (lean meat only), baked

2 or 3 cooked brussels sprouts, tossed with 3 or 4 cooked carrot coins in a sauce of:

        1 teaspoon lemon juice and a dash of dried mustard

½ cup cooked egg noodles, tossed with chopped fresh parsley

Small salad made with:

    ½ cup shredded red and white cabbage, 1 tablespoon shredded apple, and 1 teaspoon lemon juice

SNACK

    ¼ of a fresh papaya sprinkled with lime juice

DAY 6

BREAKFAST

    1 cup hot farina cereal

    2 small pitted prunes

    1 cup skim milk

LUNCH

    ¼ of a small honeydew melon, filled with:

        ¼ cup fresh or frozen raspberries and ½ cup low-fat plain yogurt

    2 squares of plain graham crackers

DINNER

Pot roast made with:

    2 ounces beef round roast, 2 tablespoons chopped onions, and ¼ cup each of turnips, parsnips, carrots, bouillon (low-salt), and wine

1 small hard roll

Small salad made with:

    1 cup romaine lettuce, 2 or 3 radishes, and 1 teaspoon lemon juice

SNACK

    ½ cup ice milk

    1 small fresh apricot

DAY 7

BREAKFAST

French toast made with:
> 1 large egg, 1 egg white, and 2 slices whole wheat bread

Blackberry syrup made of:
> 1 cup blackberries, boiled with ¼ cup water until a thick syrup is formed

1 cup skim milk

LUNCH

3 ounces roasted skinless turkey breast

5 spears (or 1 cup chopped) steamed fresh asparagus

¼ of a small baked acorn squash

Small salad made with:
> 1 cup loose-leaf lettuce, ¼ cup each of endive and cauliflower florets, and 1 tablespoon cider vinegar

SUPPER/SNACK

Salad made with:
> 1 cup each of Boston lettuce and iceberg lettuce, 2 or 3 radishes, 3 or 4 thin cucumber slices, 1 tablespoon wine vinegar, and 1 ounce blue cheese

1 small baked apple

DAY 8

BREAKFAST

1 cup cold cereal, such as corn bran

1 cup skim milk

2 small plums

LUNCH

1 sandwich made with:
> 2 slices seven-grain bread, 3 ounces water-packed tuna, and ½ cup alfalfa sprouts

1 medium orange

DINNER

¼ of a whole roasted skinless chicken

3 1-inch-diameter boiled new potatoes

1 cup steamed fresh kale

Small salad made with:
> ½ cup each of escarole and fresh spinach, ¼ cup chopped celery, and 1 teaspoon lemon juice

SNACK

10 to 12 fresh Bing cherries

DAY 9

BREAKFAST

    2 slices oatmeal bread
    ¼ cup part skim-milk ricotta cheese
    1 small Bartlett pear

LUNCH

    Salad bar salad made with:
        1 cup each of loose-leaf lettuce and
           fresh spinach; ½ cup cooked cut
           green beans; ¼ of a small avo-
           cado; ¼ cup each of chopped
           celery, mung bean sprouts, and
           diced beets; and 1 tablespoon
           cider vinegar

DINNER

    4 ounces bluefish, baked with a dash
       of dried thyme
    1 cup baked butternut squash
    2 stalks (or 1 cup chopped) steamed
       fresh broccoli
    1 small baked potato
    Small salad made with:
        1 cup red-leaf lettuce, ¼ cup water-
           cress, and 1 tablespoon lemon
           juice

SNACK

    2 spears (or ½ cup chunked) fresh
       pineapple

DAY 10

BREAKFAST

    Homemade granola made with:
        1 cup rolled oats, 1 tablespoon
           chopped almonds, 2 tablespoons
           each of shredded coconut and
           raisins, and 1 small apple, grated
    1 cup skim milk

LUNCH

    Southern-style soup made with:
        1 cup bouillon (low-salt); ¼ cup
           each of black-eyed peas, okra,
           hominy, and mustard greens; 1
           teaspoon vinegar; and a dash of
           black pepper and nutmeg
    1 small corn bread muffin*
    1 small nectarine

DINNER

    Baked stuffed zucchini made with:
        1 6 to 7-inch zucchini, chopped
           zucchini (from center of zucchini),
           ½ beaten egg, ¼ cup bread
           crumbs, and ¼ cup shredded
           cheddar cheese (low-fat,
           if possible)
    Small salad made with:
        1 cup iceberg lettuce, ½ cup curly-
           leaf lettuce, and 1 tablespoon
           vinegar

SNACK

    1 small tangerine

*Make your own, eliminating sugar and honey. To give muffin a sweet taste, mix nonfat dry milk with apple juice and use as the liquid in the recipe.

DAY 11

BREAKFAST
On a bed of lettuce, arrange:
- 1 small Red Delicious apple, sliced,
  ½ cup low-fat cottage cheese, and
  ½ cup fresh or frozen raspberries

LUNCH
Eggplant lasagna made with:
- 3 lasagna noodles, 3 slices eggplant
  (sautéed in nonstick pan), ¼ cup
  canned tomatoes with liquid,
  2 tablespoons sautéed onions and
  garlic, and ¼ teaspoon each of
  oregano and basil, topped with
  1 ounce low-fat mozzarella cheese

Small salad made with:
- 1 cup curly-leaf endive, ¼ cup
  cooked cauliflower florets, 1 teaspoon olive oil, and 1 tablespoon
  wine vinegar

DINNER
Middle-Eastern-style chicken made with:
- 3 ounces boneless, skinless
  chicken, baked in a sauce of:
  - ¼ cup low-fat plain yogurt,
    1 teaspoon lemon juice, and
    ¼ teaspoon each of turmeric
    and curry
- ½ cup steamed bulgur
- 1 cup steamed Swiss chard

Small salad made with:
- 1 cup Bibb lettuce, 3 thinly sliced
  black olives, and 3 orange sections

SNACK
- 1 small mango

DAY 12

BREAKFAST
- 2 3-inch-diameter buckwheat pancakes
- 1 cup unsweetened applesauce, heated
  with a dash of cinnamon
- 1 cup skim milk

LUNCH
On a bed of lettuce, arrange:
- ½ slice of watermelon or ⅛ of a
  medium cantaloupe or honey-
  dew melon, topped with ½ cup
  part skim-milk ricotta cheese

DINNER
- 4 ounces shad, baked with:
  - 10 white grapes and 2 tablespoons
    white wine
- ½ cup cooked pearl barley
- ½ cup cooked fresh garden peas

Small salad made with:
- ½ cup each of watercress and ice-
  berg lettuce, 1 tablespoon orange
  juice, and 1 teaspoon rosemary

SNACK
- 1 cup fresh strawberries
- ¼ cup skim milk or low-fat plain
  yogurt

DAY 13
BREAKFAST
- 1 slice whole wheat wheat berry bread
- ¼ cup low-fat cottage cheese
- 1 small D'Anjou pear

LUNCH
- 1 sandwich made with:
  - 2 slices whole wheat bread, ½ cup crabmeat, ¼ cup mung bean sprouts, and 2 leaves Boston lettuce
- 1 small Red Delicious apple

DINNER
Middle-Eastern meal made with:
- 1 whole wheat pita pocket bread, stuffed with a sauté of:
  - ½ cup mashed garbanzo beans;
  - 1 small tomato, chopped;
  - 2 garlic cloves, crushed;
  - ¼ teaspoon each of cumin and saffron; and topped with
  - ¼ cup low-fat plain yogurt
- Baba Ghannouj made with:
  - ½ cup boiled eggplant; 1 teaspoon each of lemon juice, fresh cilantro (or coriander), and garlic powder; and 1 tablespoon tahini (sesame seed paste)*

SNACK
Berry shake made with:
- 1 cup skim milk and ½ cup frozen berries, blended in a blender

DAY 14
BREAKFAST
- 1 cup hot whole wheat cereal
- 1 cup skim milk
- ¼ of a fresh papaya, sprinkled with lime juice

LUNCH
- 1 sandwich made with:
  - 2 slices oatmeal-raisin bread, 2 teaspoons peanut butter*, and topped with ½ small banana, sliced
- 1 cup skim milk
- 1 small peach

DINNER
Chinese stir fry made with:
- 3 ounces pork shoulder (lean meat only), 1 cup shredded cabbage, 2 tablespoons chopped onions, and ¼ cup chopped celery
- ½ cup cooked brown rice
- ½ cup snow peas sautéed with:
  - 2 tablespoons chopped straw-type mushrooms and 1 tablespoon chopped cashew nuts

SNACK
- 2 small plums

*Tahini is available in natural foods stores, specialty food shops, and some supermarkets.

*Buy peanut butter without sugar and salt, if possible.

DAY 15
BREAKFAST
    2 slices nine-grain bread
    1 ounce Muenster cheese
    2 spears (or ½ cup chunked) fresh
       pineapple

LUNCH
Salad made with:
       1 cup spinach; ¼ cup each of
          shredded carrots, sliced
          cucumbers, chopped green
          peppers, and sliced radishes; and
       1 tablespoon wine vinegar
    1 small whole wheat roll
    1 small persimmon or fresh fruit in
       season

DINNER
Mexican tostada made with:
    1 corn tortilla filled with:
       ½ cup each of pinto beans and
          shredded iceberg lettuce,
          ¼ cup each of shredded
          Monterey Jack cheese and
          chopped tomatoes, and hot
          salsa to taste
    2 or 3 slivers raw jicama

SNACK
    ½ of a small banana, sliced in half and
       baked with:
       1 teaspoon each of raisins and
          chopped filbert nuts

DAY 16
BREAKFAST
    1 cup dry cereal, such as 100 percent
       bran
    1 cup skim milk
    ½ of a medium grapefruit

LUNCH
    1 sandwich made with
       2 slices pumpernickel bread,
          1 ounce Brie or Camembert,
          ½ cup alfalfa sprouts, 2 or 3
          cauliflower florets, and 3 or 4
          radishes, sliced
10 to 12 Emperor grapes

DINNER
    4 ounces trout, poached in:
       2 tablespoons buttermilk and
       ⅛ teaspoon dillweed
    ½ cup cooked wild and brown rice,
       mixed
5 or 6 spears (or 1 cup chopped)
       cooked white asparagus
Small salad made with:
    1 cup spinach, ¼ cup each of sliced
       raw zucchini and grated raw sweet
       potato, and 1 tablespoon lemon
       juice

SNACK
    1 cup low-fat plain yogurt
    ½ cup cubed casaba melon

DAY 17

BREAKFAST

- 1 large egg, poached or boiled
- 1 slice oatmeal-nut or whole wheat bread
- 1 small orange

LUNCH

A country kettle-style soup made with:

- 1 cup dark greens (Swiss chard, bok choy, kale, or spinach); ¼ cup each of Great Northern beans, shredded carrots, and chopped celery; 2 tablespoons chopped onions, and ½ cup bouillon (low-salt)
- 2 rye crackers
- 1 slice of watermelon

DINNER

Tofu stir-fry made with:

- 1 2- by 2-inch square of tofu; ½ cup each of chopped celery and mung bean sprouts; ¼ cup each of chopped sweet red peppers, chopped green peppers, bamboo shoots, and water chestnuts; 1 tablespoon chopped ginger root; and 2 tablespoons soy sauce (low-salt)
- ½ cup cooked brown rice

SNACK

- 1 medium tangerine
- 1 ounce cheddar cheese (low-fat, if possible)

DAY 18

BREAKFAST

- 1 cup hot whole wheat cereal
- 2 medium stewed prunes
- 1 cup skim milk

LUNCH

On a plate arrange:

- ½ each of a medium apple, pear, and orange; ¼ cup grapefruit sections; and top with ¼ cup low-fat plain yogurt flavored with a drop of vanilla extract
- 1 small roll or 1 slice whole wheat bread
- 1 cup skim milk

DINNER

- ½ of a whole baked skinless chicken breast
- ½ cup cooked spinach noodles
- ½ cup cooked brussels sprouts
- 1 cup mashed pumpkin

Small salad made with:

- 1 cup Bibb lettuce; ¼ small tomato, sliced; and 1 tablespoon low-calorie French dressing

SNACK

Berry shake made with:

- 1 cup skim milk or low-fat buttermilk and 1 cup frozen berries, blended in a blender

DAY 19

BREAKFAST

1 4-inch-square waffle

Peach conserve, made of:

    1 medium peach, sliced and boiled in a little water until a thick conserve or syrup is formed

1 cup skim milk

LUNCH

Cottage cheese dip made with:

    ¼ cup low-fat cottage cheese and a dash each of dillweed, black pepper, and lemon juice

5 or 6 cucumber spears

1 stalk celery

1 stalk broccoli

2 or 3 cauliflower florets

1 medium Golden Delicious apple

DINNER

Bean loaf made with:

    ½ cup drained kidney beans, 1 ounce shredded cheddar cheese (low-fat, if possible), 2 tablespoons chopped onions, ¼ cup each of chopped celery and bread crumbs, and ½ cup beaten egg

1 cup steamed zucchini

Small salad made with:

    1 cup Boston lettuce, ¼ cup each of watercress and bean sprouts, and 1 tablespoon lemon juice

SNACK

2 medium plums

DAY 20

BREAKFAST

1 cup hot whole wheat cereal

1 cup skim milk

2 kiwi fruits

LUNCH

1 sandwich made with:

    2 slices caraway rye bread, 3 ounces water-packed tuna, 1 ounce Swiss cheese, 2 or 3 tomato slices, and 1 lettuce leaf

1 medium tangelo or orange

DINNER

A shepherd's-style stew made with:

    2 ounces lamb shoulder (lean meat only), ½ cup each of peas and carrots, 2 tablespoons chopped onions, and topped with dumplings made of:

        ½ cup flour, ½ teaspoon baking powder, 3 tablespoons skim milk, and 1 teaspoon safflower oil

Small salad made with:

    1 cup endive, ½ cup spinach, and 1 tablespoon wine vinegar

SNACK

¼ of a small casaba melon

DAY 21

BREAKFAST

    1 cup oatmeal, cooked with 2 table-
       spoons raisins

    1 cup skim milk

LUNCH

    A Greek salad made with:

        1 cup spinach, 4 or 5 cucumber
           slices, ¼ cup shredded carrots,
           2 or 3 green olives, 1 ounce feta
           cheese, and 1 tablespoon bal-
           samic or wine vinegar

    1 whole wheat pita pocket bread

    1 small orange

DINNER

    Foiled fish made with:

   4 to 5 ounces white fish, 1 tablespoon
         white wine, and 1 teaspoon basil,
         baked in aluminum foil

    1 cup cooked green beans

    ½ cup mashed turnips

    Small salad made with:

        1 cup red-leaf lettuce, ¼ cup grated
           daikon radish*, and 1 tablespoon
           wine vinegar

SNACK

    Apple crisp made with:

        ½ of a small apple, thinly sliced,
           and topped with:

           ¼ cup rolled oats, 1 tablespoon
              raisins, 1 teaspoon honey,
              and 2 teaspoons chopped
              walnuts

*A large white radish available at many grocery stores and
green grocers.

Sources of Nutrients in the Turn-Back-the-Clock Diet

Nutrient	Sources	Nutrient	Sources
CARBOHY-DRATES	Bread Candy Cereal grains Corn Dried peas and beans Fruits Jelly Milk Pastas Vegetables	Iron	Dark green leafy vegetables Dried fruits (raisins, prunes) Dried peas and beans Egg yolks Kidneys Liver Red meat Whole grain and enriched breads and cereals
FATS	Butter Cheese Cream Egg yolks Margarine Meat and the fat around it Oil Peanut butter Salad dressing Shortening Whole milk	Magnesium	Dark green leafy vegetables Legumes Nuts Seeds
PROTEIN	Cheese Dried peas and beans Eggs Fish Legumes Lentils Meat Milk Nuts Poultry Seeds	Phosphorus	Eggs Fish Legumes Meat Milk and milk products Nuts Poultry
		Potassium	Bananas Bran Dried fruits Dried peas and beans Orange juice Peanut butter
MINERALS Calcium	Dark green leafy vegetables Milk and milk products Canned fish with bones Tofu	Selenium	Egg yolks Meat Milk Poultry Seafood Whole grain products
Iodine	Iodized salt Saltwater fish Sea salt	Zinc	Eggs Liver Meat Seafood

Nutrient	Sources	Nutrient	Sources
VITAMINS		*Vitamin B$_{12}$*	Eggs
Vitamin A	Apricots	*(Cobalamin)*	Fish
	Broccoli		Meat
	Cantaloupe		Milk and milk products
	Carrots		Poultry
	Dark green leafy vegetables		(Not present in plant foods)
	Fish-liver oil		
	Liver	*Folate*	Dark green leafy vegetables
	Milk	*(folic acid)*	Dried peas and beans
	Peaches		Liver
	Sweet potatoes		Wheat germ
	Winter squash		
		Vitamin C	Broccoli
B Vitamins		(ascorbic	Cabbage
Vitamin B$_1$	Cashews	acid)	Cantaloupe
(Thiamine)	Dried peas and beans		Citrus fruits
	Liver		Dark green leafy vegetables
	Pork		Green peppers
	Whole grain and enriched		Potatoes
	breads and cereals		Strawberries
Vitamin B$_2$	Dark green leafy vegetables	Vitamin D	Butter
(Riboflavin)	Dried peas and beans		Eggs
	Liver		Fortified milk
	Milk and milk products		Liver
	Whole grain breads		Margarine
	and cereals		Saltwater fish and their oils
Niacin	Fish		
	Liver	Vitamin E	Fats and polyunsaturated
	Meat		oils of vegetable products
	Whole grain and enriched		Seeds
	breads, cereals, and pastas		Whole grains
Vitamin B$_6$	Bananas		
(Pyridoxine)	Liver	Vitamin K	Cabbage
	Meats		Green leafy vegetables
	Nuts and seeds		Liver
	Poultry		Peas
	Whole grain breads, cereals,		Potatoes
	and pastas		

Caloric Content of Some Common Foods

Food	Amount	Calories
Beverages		
Alcoholic		
Beer	12 ounces	151
Whiskey, gin, rum, vodka, etc.		
80 proof	1½ ounces	97
86 proof	1½ ounces	105
Wine		
Dessert	3½ ounces	141
Table	3½ ounces	87
Fruit drinks and juices		
Apple juice	6 ounces	87
Apricot nectar	6 ounces	107
Cocoa, in 1 cup water	1 ounce	102
Cranberry juice cocktail	6 ounces	124
Grape juice	6 ounces	125
Lemonade	6 ounces	81
Orange juice	6 ounces	84
Prune juice	6 ounces	148
Soda		
Club	12 ounces	0
Cola	12 ounces	144
Cream	12 ounces	160
Fruit-flavored	12 ounces	171
Ginger ale	12 ounces	113
Tonic	12 ounces	113
Vegetable juices		
Tomato juice cocktail	6 ounces	38
Vegetable juice cocktail	6 ounces	31
Breads		
Biscuits	2	206
Boston brown bread	1 slice	95
Crackers		
Butter	5	87
Cheese	10	150

Food	Amount	Calories
Cheese-peanut butter sandwiches	4	139
Graham	1	55
Rye wafers	5	112
Saltines	4	48
Italian	1 slice	56
Muffins, blueberry	1	112
Pancakes, from mix, with milk and eggs	1 (6 in. diameter)	164
Pizza, with cheese topping	1 slice	153
Pretzels, thin	5	117
Rolls, hard	1	156
Rye	1 slice	61
Stuffing, bread	½ cup	208
Waffles, from mix, with milk and eggs	1 (7 in. diameter)	206
White	1 slice	76
Whole wheat	1 slice	67
Condiments		
Jams and preserves	1 tablespoon	54
Marmalade	1 tablespoon	51
Mayonnaise	1 tablespoon	101
Olives, mission	5 large	44
Salad dressing, commercial	1 tablespoon	66
Sauerkraut	½ cup	21
Dairy Foods		
Cheeses		
Blue or Roquefort	1 ounce	104
Camembert	1 ounce	85
Cheddar	1 ounce	113
Cottage, creamed	6 ounces	180
Swiss	1 ounce	104

Food	Amount	Calories
Cream		
Sour, cultured	1 tablespoon	25
Sweet	1 tablespoon	32
Whipped	1 tablespoon	27
Ice cream, vanilla	½ cup	127
Milk, whole	6 ounces	119
Yogurt, low-fat, plain	1 cup	113

Desserts

Food	Amount	Calories
Cakes		
Chocolate, with icing	1 small piece	277
Fruitcake	1 slice (1 ounce)	114
Gingerbread	1 piece (3 × 3 × 2 in.)	371
Pound cake	1 slice (1 ounce)	142
Sponge cake	1 slice (2 ounces)	196
Cookies		
Assorted	6	250
Brownies, with nuts	1 (3 × 3 × 1 in.)	97
Chocolate chip	1	51
Fig bars	1	50
Gingersnaps	1	29
Macaroons	1	90
Marshmallow	1	74
Oatmeal, with raisins	1	59
Oreo-type	1	50
Raisin, biscuit-type	1	67
Sugar wafers	1 large	44
Vanilla wafers	1 large	19
Cream puffs, filled	1	303
Custard, baked	1 cup	305
Doughnuts	1	164
Gelatin dessert, made with water	1 cup	142

Food	Amount	Calories
Pies		
Apple	1 piece (⅛ pie)	302
Banana custard	1 piece (⅛ pie)	252
Blueberry	1 piece (⅛ pie)	286
Boston cream	1 piece (⅛ pie)	208
Coconut custard	1 piece (⅛ pie)	268
Lemon meringue	1 piece (⅛ pie)	268
Mince	1 piece (⅛ pie)	320
Pecan	1 piece (⅙ pie)	431
Pumpkin	1 piece (⅛ pie)	241
Puddings		
Bread, with raisins	½ cup	248
Chocolate	½ cup	193
Rice, with raisins	½ cup	194
Tapioca cream	½ cup	111

Eggs

Food	Amount	Calories
Hard-cooked	1 large	82

Fats and Oils

Food	Amount	Calories
Butter	1 teaspoon	36
Margarine	1 teaspoon	36
Oils, vegetable	1 tablespoon	120

Fish (see also Shellfish)

Food	Amount	Calories
Bluefish, broiled or baked with butter	6 ounces	270
Fish sticks, breaded	6 ounces	300
Flounder, baked with butter	6 ounces	342
Halibut, broiled with butter	6 ounces	288

(continued)

Caloric Content of Some Common Foods—*Continued*

Food	Amount	Calories
Fish (*continued*)		
Salmon		
Baked, with butter	6 ounces	312
Sockeye, canned	3 ounces	145
Sardines, canned		
(drained)	1 can	187
Tuna, canned		
Oil-packed		
Drained	6½ ounces	309
With oil	6½ ounces	530
Water-packed	6½ ounces	234
Fruits		
Apples	1 medium-size	80
Applesauce	½ cup	116
Apricots		
Fresh	3	55
Dried	¼ cup	85
Avocados	½	188
Bananas	1	101
Blueberries		
Fresh	½ cup	45
Frozen, sweetened	½ cup	121
Cherries, fresh	10	47
Citrus		
Grapefruit	½	40
Oranges	1	65
Tangerines	1	46
Dates	5	110
Grapes, seedless	10	34
Mangoes	1	152
Muskmelons		
Cantaloupe	½	82
Casaba	1 wedge	38
	(1/10 melon)	
Honeydew	1 wedge	49
	(1/10 melon)	
Nectarines	1	88
Peaches		
Fresh	1	58
Dried	5 large	190
	halves	

Food	Amount	Calories
Pears, Bartlett	1	100
Pineapple		
Fresh	2 slices	88
Canned, with syrup	2 slices	156
Plums	1	32
Prunes	5	137
Raisins	⅓ cup	124
Watermelon	1 wedge	111
	(4 in. thick)	
Grains and Grain Products		
Brown rice, cooked	½ cup	116
Cornmeal, degermed,		
cooked	3½ ounces	50
Oatmeal, cooked	1 cup	132
Wheat bran	1 ounce	60
Wheat germ, toasted	6 tablespoons	138
Legumes		
Dried beans		
Mung, sprouted	1 cup	37
Navy		
Baked, Boston-style,		
with pork	1 cup	311
Cooked	1 cup	224
Soybeans		
Cooked	1 cup	234
Tofu	1 piece	86
	(2½ × 2¾ × 1 in.)	
Lentils, cooked	1 cup	212
Peanuts		
Peanut butter	1 tablespoon	94
Roasted in shell	10	105
Peas		
Black-eyed, cooked	1 cup	174
Split, cooked	1 cup	232

Caloric Content of Some Common Foods—*Continued*

Food	Amount	Calories	Food	Amount	Calories
Meats*			Heart		
			Beef, braised	6 ounces	323
Beef			Calf, braised	6 ounces	354
Corned	3 ounces	316	Liver		
Ground			Beef, fried	6 ounces	390
Lean	3 ounces	185	Calf, fried	6 ounces	448
Regular	3 ounces	245	Poultry, simmered	6 ounces	283
Pot roast			Sweetbreads,		
Lean and fat	6 ounces	490	calf, braised	6 ounces	288
Lean only	5 ounces	280	Tongue, beef,		
Rib roast			braised	6 ounces	415
Lean and fat	6 ounces	750	Tripe	6 ounces	220
Lean only	5.4 ounces	375			
Steak					
Round, broiled			**Nuts and Seeds**		
Lean and fat	6 ounces	440			
Lean only	4.8 ounces	260	Almonds	about 11	85
Sirloin, broiled			Brazil nuts	6 large	185
Lean and fat	6 ounces	660	Cashews, roasted in	about 14	159
Lean only	4 ounces	230	oil	large	
Lamb chops, lean	2	280	Pecans	10 halves	124
	(5.2 ounces)		Pumpkin seeds	1 ounce	157
			Sesame seeds	1 ounce	161
Pork			Sunflower seeds	1 ounce	100
Bacon	2 slices	86	Walnuts, English	14 halves	185
Chops, lean and fat	2 thick	520			
	(3.5 ounces				
	each)		**Pasta**		
Ham			Macaroni, with cheese	1 cup	430
Boiled	2 ounces	135	Noodles	½ cup	100
Cured, lean and fat	6 ounces	490	Spaghetti,		
Roast, lean and fat	6 ounces	620	with meatballs,		
Sausage	1 patty	129	tomato sauce, and		
	(2 ounces		Parmesan cheese	1 cup	332
	before				
	cooking)				
Veal			**Poultry and Game**		
Cutlet, medium fat	6 ounces	370			
Roast, medium fat	6 ounces	460	Chicken		
Luncheon meats			Chicken à la king	1 cup	468
Bologna	2 ounces	170	Chicken and		
Liverwurst	3 ounces	265	noodles	1 cup	367
Salami	3 ounces	145	Chicken fricassee	1 cup	386
Variety meats			Fried (including	½ breast,	335
Gizzard, chicken,			bone)	2 drumsticks	
simmered	6 ounces	253		(7.5 ounces)	

*All meat values are for cooked meat

(continued)

Caloric Content of Some Common Foods—*Continued*

Food	Amount	Calories	Food	Amount	Calories
Poultry and Game *(continued)*			Beets, cooked	1 cup	218
			Broccoli, cooked	1 cup	40
Chicken *(continued)*			Brussels sprouts,		
Roasted, flesh, skin,			cooked	½ cup	28
and giblets	½ pound	549	Cabbage, cooked	1 cup	31
Roasted,			Carrots		
white meat only	½ pound	413	Raw	1	30
Duck, roasted,			Cooked, sliced	½ cup	24
flesh and skin	6 ounces	558	Cauliflower, cooked	½ cup	14
Goose, roasted,			Celery	1 large stalk	7
flesh and skin	6 ounces	756	Corn		
Rabbit, stewed, flesh	6 ounces	371	Cooked on the cob	1 ear	70
Turkey, roasted,			Canned	½ cup	70
white and dark			Cucumbers	1 small	25
meat	6 ounces	324	Eggplant,		
			cooked, diced	1 cup	38
Shellfish *(see also* Fish*)*			Kale, cooked	½ cup	22
			Lettuce	1 head	72
Crab, deviled	1 cup	451	Mushrooms, sliced	½ cup	10
Lobster, cooked	1 cup	138	Onions, sliced	¼ cup	11
Oysters, raw	3 ounces	57	Peas, cooked	⅓ cup	41
Scallops,			Peppers, green	1 large	36
breaded and fried	6⅔ ounces	367	Potatoes		
Shrimp, french-fried	3 ounces	192	Baked	1 large	145
			French fried	10 (4 in. long)	214
Sweeteners			Mashed, with milk		
			and butter	½ cup	99
Honey	1 tablespoon	64	Radishes	5 medium-	4
Molasses, blackstrap	1 tablespoon	43		size	
Sugar, granulated	1 tablespoon	48	Spinach, cooked	1 cup	41
Syrups, table blend	1 tablespoon	60	Squash, summer,		
			cooked	1 cup	25
Vegetables			Tomatoes	1	40
			Turnips, cooked,		
Asparagus, cooked	4 spears	12	cubed	½ cup	18
Beans, cooked			Vegetables, mixed	½ cup	58
Green	1 cup	31	Watercress	1 cup	7
Lima	1 cup	189			

ANTI-
AGING
EXERCISES

Chapter 2

A couple of years ago after I'd started working out with weights, I decided, "If I can do this, I can jog, too." So I tried jogging—initially in the wrong shoes and my husband's old gray sweatsuit. I tried it for two days. I huffed and puffed—jogging hurt. I wore a watch and kept glancing at it. It seemed as though those 15 minutes would never end. The first day, I started walking 13½ minutes after I'd started. I felt hot, flushed, sweaty, out-of-breath . . . and yet, a strange sensation had come over me. I inhaled and realized that I had been taking the deepest breaths I'd ever taken in my life. Oxygen seemed to have penetrated every tired bone and joint, bringing each one back to life. And my head—I felt as though years of dust and cobwebs had been swept away; my brain felt cleansed and rejuvenated, ready to see me through reading a volume of Plato, solving a family crisis, surviving a tough day at the office, or facing any challenge that life might present. On the second day a neighbor saw me staggering and panting to get to my door and said, "Donna, are you mad?"

"I do this because it feels so good when I stop!" I replied.

I liked the way my body took in all that oxygen and left me feeling both calm and energetic at the same time, so much that I invested in proper shoes and a flag-red jogging suit. I began running almost every day. On the days I didn't run, I didn't feel right. The cobwebs stayed in my head, and I felt irritable. On the days I did run, I felt happy. Even when things weren't really going so well, the extra oxygen I'd taken in seemed to have a way of penetrating deep, pleasant interiors of my memory, pulling out silly things my sisters and I had done together when we were little or pleasant moments when my husband and I had first met. At the risk of looking like some kind of grinning fool, I let myself feel elated even when there was no apparent reason for it. I slept well, too, and began to remember my dreams more vividly. I knew that something strange and wonderful had happened to me on the night I dreamed that I was flapping my arms, inhaling fresh, heavenly oxygen, and soaring over New York City. As I flew, that same neighbor stared up at me from the ground in astonishment and said, "Donna, are you mad? You can't fly!" I had been converted. I was an exercise addict.

Only one thing was missing. The next day I went out and bought a Walkman radio and cassette player so that I could have music when I jogged. I was actually looking forward to the process of exercising, gliding through the fresh air, witnessing the first buds of spring and the crisp early foliage of autumn, with Beethoven or Bruce Springsteen at my side.

Eventually, I got tired of running every day, and besides, I felt the toll on my knees and ankles, so I began to alternate running with

Lynn Sherman, 49: Runner

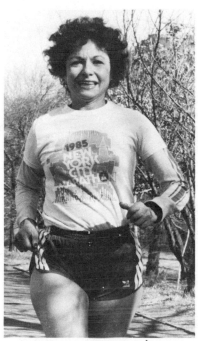

"I'm a devoted runner, but I wasn't always like this. When I was 41 and my boyfriend suggested that I try running, I shrieked at him, 'Running? I don't even like to walk!' But I started, running just a mile or two at first—and this year I ran my first marathon. Running has taken inches off my entire frame and given me lean muscle instead of fat. Psychologically I feel much better, and I have a sort of discipline I never had before that carries over into all aspects of life. I'm amazed at myself—I run six days a week, from 6:30 to 7:00 A.M., before going to work. I've become very diet conscious, too. When I was getting ready for the marathon, I went on a largely carbohydrate diet, eating plenty of rice, pasta, legumes, and fruit. I'm a person who can gain weight just by looking at food, so I continue to live mostly on small portions of complex carbohydrates. The diet helps me run, and running helps me live!"

dancing classes. But dancing still jarred my joints somewhat. So I decided to try swimming, and now I belong to the Vanderbilt Y in midtown Manhattan, and every day I either swim, take an exercise class, work out with weights, or run (but now I warm up properly before I start, an important step I had missed in my original running program—and a kindness to my knees and ankles).

My routine is no routine at all, so I never get bored with exercise. I actually look forward to my daily 30 to 45 minutes of working out, when I can put all other thoughts out of my mind and pamper my mind, body, and spirit. How do I find time? Since I spend less time sleeping, the time to exercise is there for me to use. But then I'm an addict. Incidentally,

The Ideal Way to Your Ideal Weight
through Aerobic Exercise

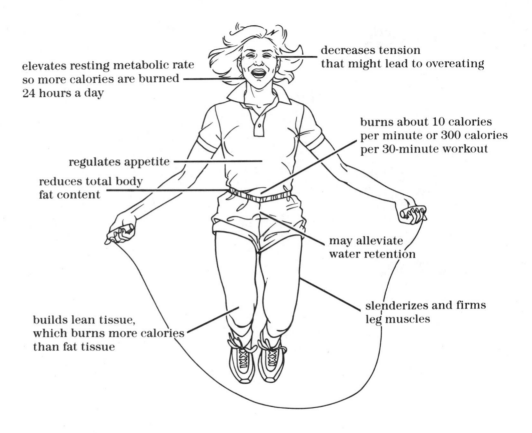

elevates resting metabolic rate
so more calories are burned
24 hours a day

decreases tension
that might lead to overeating

burns about 10 calories
per minute or 300 calories
per 30-minute workout

regulates appetite

reduces total body
fat content

may alleviate
water retention

slenderizes and firms
leg muscles

builds lean tissue,
which burns more calories
than fat tissue

I've lost a couple of inches from my waist and an inch from my upper arms since I started exercising. I hardly ever get sick or even catch a cold, and sex is better than ever.

But I don't try to force exercise on my friends or family. They would only laugh at me and tell me I'm a fanatic. However, when they ask me how I got these toned-up muscles and the glow in my complexion, I smile to myself as I answer, "Oh, I work at it."

Of course, if I want to feel terrific for the rest of my life, I'll have to keep up this anti-aging maneuver. That's why it's so important to pick exercises that you enjoy, and be so serious about doing them that when you travel, you take along the jogging shoes, the jump rope, the tennis racquet—or whatever equipment you need to keep up the good work.

It would be nice to have Romana Kryzanowska's animated zest and joie de vivre just by wishing, but Romana, the director of the Isotonic (the Pilates Method) Exercise Studio in New York City, stays in her prime with regular exercise and teaches her clients to do so as well. This is what she has to say: "Combating the effects of aging is combating gravity. You have to keep good posture and keep tall. Without exercise, our backs and our muscles go after 40. It's so important to have proper exercise, not strenuous exercise, but proper. It gets the blood circulating to our joints and through the capillaries down to our fingertips. Exercise creates energy and energy makes you capable of doing more."

Women have known the value of exercise for a long time; it has just taken them a while to do anything about it en masse. The feminists of the late nineteenth and early twentieth centuries recognized that the ideal Victorian woman—pale, languorous, and suffering frequent fainting spells and bouts of hysteria—was a product of a society that demanded she virtually paralyze herself with constricting corsets and a life devoid of mental or physical activity. As early as 1853, Madame Lola Montez, the famous nineteenth-century courtesan and dancer, gave this advice in her book *The Arts and Secrets of Beauty:* "The first thing to be thought of is health, for there can be no development of beauty in sickly fibres. Plenty of exercise, in the open air, is the great recipe.... A bent and stooping form is quite sure to come of a bent and stooping spirit...."

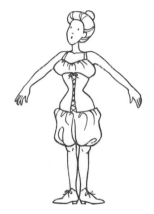

Fortunately for us, during our lifetime women have loosened the binds, shed girdles (Remember girdles?), and made foot-pampering tennis and jogging shoes fashionable. No one minds if you come for Sunday brunch in a jogging suit and a touch of eau de sweat. They just envy the way you can scarf down two whole wheat carrot muffins and look so trim.

SHAPING UP

It isn't a magic potion that works overnight, but exercise is the one *dependable* way to burn off calories and keep them from coming back. If you keep it up, exercise will speed up your metabolism so that you can eat more, if you feel inclined to eat more, and stay trim.

The accompanying table shows how many calories you burn in an hour of various activities, depending on your weight. As you'll see, burning anywhere from 70 to 500 calories an hour for several hours a week will help you to slim down in no time. Of course, exercise does more than melt away pounds. Its main purpose is to condition your body.

Activity Calorie Chart

Calories Burned in 1 Hour
Body Weight (in pounds)

Activity	105-126	127-148	149-170	171-192	193-214
Badminton					
Singles (recreational)	275-295	310-330	350-370	385-405	425
Doubles (recreational)	235-250	270-285	300-315	335-350	365
Bicycling, 10 mph	325-350	370-395	415-440	460-475	505
Bowling—regular	150-160	170-180	190-200	210-220	230
Calisthenics					
Medium	350-370	395-420	445-470	490-515	540
High	435-465	495-525	555-585	615-645	675
Playing cards	70-75	80-85	90-95	100-105	110
Playing chess	70-75	80-85	90-95	100-105	110
Dancing					
Aerobic—medium	350-370	395-420	445-470	490-515	540
Aerobic—high	515-550	585-620	655-690	725-760	795
Square	330-350	375-400	420-445	465-480	510
Polka	425-455	480-510	540-570	600-630	655
Waltz	195-210	225-240	250-265	280-295	305
Preparing dinner	105-110	120-125	135-140	150-155	160
Driving a car					
Automatic—light traffic	75-80	85-90	95-100	105-110	115
Automatic—heavy traffic	80-85	90-95	100-105	110-115	120
Standard—light traffic	80-85	90-95	100-105	110-115	120
Standard—heavy traffic	105-110	120-125	135-140	150-155	160
Eating	70-75	80-85	90-95	100-105	110
Gardening	305-325	345-365	390-410	430-450	470
Golf (foursome, 9 holes in					
2 hours, pulling clubs)	195-210	225-240	250-265	280-295	305
Gymnastics					
Light	235-250	270-285	300-315	335-350	365
Medium	400-430	455-485	510-540	565-595	620
Hard	555-595	635-670	710-750	785-825	865
Hiking					
20-pound pack, 2 mph	235-250	270-285	300-315	335-350	365
20-pound pack, 4 mph	355-375	400-425	450-475	500-525	550
Housework					
Light	160-170	180-195	205-215	225-235	250
Strenuous	195-210	225-240	250-265	280-295	305
Horseback riding					
Walk	130-140	150-155	165-175	185-195	205
Trot	325-350	370-395	415-440	460-475	505
Gallop	470-500	535-565	600-630	665-695	730
Jogging					
11-minute mile, 5.5 mph	515-550	585-620	655-690	725-760	795
8½-minute mile, 7.2 mph	550-585	625-660	700-735	775-810	850

Activity	Calories Burned in 1 Hour Body Weight (in pounds)				
	105–126	127–148	149–170	171–192	193–214
Martial arts	620-660	705-750	790-835	875-920	960
Mowing lawn—push	360-385	410-435	460-485	510-535	560
Mowing lawn—power	195-210	225-240	250-265	280-295	305
Office work—secretarial	115-120	130-135	145-150	160-170	175
Playing the piano	95-100	110-115	120-130	135-140	150
Personal grooming (dressing, washing, showering)	160-170	180-195	205-215	225-235	250
Raking leaves	175-185	200-210	220-235	245-260	270
Reading	70-75	80-85	90-95	100-105	110
Rowing					
2 mph	235-250	270-285	300-315	335-350	365
4 mph	515-550	585-620	655-690	725-760	795
Running in place					
50-60 steps per minute (counting one foot only)	400-430	455-485	510-540	565-595	620
70-80 steps per minute (counting one foot only)	435-465	495-525	555-585	615-645	675
90-100 steps per minute (counting one foot only)	515-550	585-620	655-690	725-760	795
Sailing					
Calm water	120-130	140-145	155-165	170-180	190
Rough water	145-155	165-175	185-195	205-215	225
Scuba diving	355-375	400-425	450-475	500-525	550
Sex					
Foreplay	80-85	90-95	100-105	110-115	120
Intercourse					
Submissive role	105-110	120-125	135-140	150-155	160
Aggressive role	235-250	270-285	300-315	335-350	365
Shopping	130-140	150-155	165-175	185-195	205
Skating (ice and roller)					
Light	275-295	310-330	350-370	385-405	425
Vigorous	485-520	555-590	620-655	690-720	755
Skiing					
Downhill	465-500	530-560	595-625	660-690	720
Cross country, 5 mph	550-585	625-660	700-735	775-810	850
Water	375-405	430-455	480-505	535-560	585
Skipping rope					
50-60 skips per minute (counting one foot only)	400-430	455-485	510-540	565-595	620
70-80 skips per minute (counting one foot only)	435-465	495-525	555-585	615-645	675
90-100 skips per minute (counting one foot only)	515-550	585-620	655-690	725-760	795

(continued)

Activity Calorie Chart—*Continued*

Calories Burned in 1 Hour
Body Weight (in pounds)

Activity	105–126	127–148	149–170	171–192	193–214
Sledding	335-355	380-405	425-450	470-495	520
Sleeping	50-55	60	65-70	75-80	80
Standing (without activity)	80-85	90-95	100-105	110-115	120
Stationary bicycling					
Pulse rate to 130, 10 mph	330-355	375-400	420-445	465-490	515
Pulse rate to 130, 15 mph	515-550	585-620	655-690	725-760	795
Pulse rate to 130, 20 mph	700-745	795-840	885-935	985-1,030	1,080
Swimming					
Crawl—20 yards per minute	235-250	270-285	300-315	335-350	365
Crawl—30 yards per minute	330-350	375-400	420-445	465-480	510
Crawl—45 yards per minute	540-575	615-650	690-725	765-800	835
Table tennis	235-250	270-285	300-315	335-350	365
Tennis					
Singles (recreational)	335-355	380-405	425-450	470-495	520
Doubles (recreational)	235-250	270-285	300-315	335-350	365
Volleyball (recreational)	275-295	310-330	350-370	385-405	425
Waitressing	190-205	215-230	245-255	270-285	295
Walking					
2 mph	145-155	165-175	185-195	205-215	225
3 mph	235-250	270-285	300-315	335-350	365
5 mph	435-465	495-525	555-585	615-645	675
Washing dishes	105-110	120-125	135-140	150-155	160
Watching TV	60-65	70-75	80	85-90	95
Weight training	235-250	270-285	300-315	335-350	365
Writing	70-75	80-85	90-95	100-105	110
Yoga	180-195	205-220	230-245	255-270	280

SOURCE: Charles T. Kuntzleman, *Maximum Personal Energy* (Emmaus, Pa.: Rodale Press, 1984).

THE BENEFITS OF EXERCISING

A fit-looking body depends on the good health of 696 different muscles. If these muscles are all firm and resilient, you'll have a figure that stops traffic. Without exercise, the muscles will let things sag, so we all develop fat and flab in our own individual trouble spots—arms, waist, stomach, hips, thighs, or all of the above.

If you're overweight, you'll want to start with aerobic exercise to melt the pounds. Simply taking a brisk, 20-minute walk every other day can burn off several pounds of fat per year. You can speed up the process with more strenuous aerobics—race-walking, swimming, bicycling, cross-country skiing, running, or such for 20 to 30 minutes at a time, three or four times a week.

Depending on the exercise you choose, aerobics also improve your strength and endurance and exercise the heart, your most important muscle. To keep up your muscles' stamina, however, you might want to vary your routine with weight lifting or calisthenics workouts. If your weight is average, exercise might not show its effect in missing pounds because you'll be building up muscles that weigh more than fat. But take a tape measure, and judge the results by inches. Buy a gorgeous belt that's just a little too tight—then try it on two months after you've started a faithful exercise program. That's where the rewards become evident.

Even if you're a slender, delicate type, stop listening to people who tell you, "Oh, you don't need to exercise, you wispy dear." Wait until you see what exercise can do for you. You'll look good in a bathing suit again; you'll lose any middle-aged paunch you've developed, and you'll be able to tote your own 75 pounds of luggage, so that you'll never again have to play the helpless woman, unless you want to.

EXERCISE AND MOOD

"When the going gets tough, the tough go to the gym," is my friend Alice's motto. She swears that exercise kept her from knuckling under a few years ago when she found herself divorced and trying to support herself and two teenagers. All of her friends wondered how she managed to look fresh and serene, her sense of humor intact, even though she was working long hours in a demanding but unrewarding job. "Whenever I had a moment, I sneaked off to the nearby Y for a swim, jogged, or worked out on my exercycle at home," she says. "It was the best investment of a little time and money I ever made." She says exercise gave her the energy to go back to school while working and the enthusiasm to find a better job and eventually a better mate.

Clinical researchers have a number of theories as to why exercise beats away the blues. Just consider the nature of depression. Psychologists call it anger turned inward, made passive. Depression is more common in women than in men; no one knows why. We do know that activity itself is one way to alleviate depression. Add to that the enhanced body image that you get every time you look at your improved figure in the mirror—another sure way to ward off feelings of despair. Exercise can also boost your mood because of the sense of self-mastery you get after a workout. And don't discount the cathartic outlet provided by exercise for pent-up anxiety and anger. However, fitness specialists also

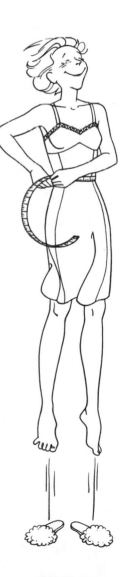

Reducing Flab

The only way to burn away fat is with aerobic exercise, but if you want to tone your muscles, you might want to work out with weights several times a week to supplement your aerobic workouts.

"To tighten muscles is hard but not impossible," says Carl Lubet, New York City weight trainer. "It takes three to six weeks to toughen the connective tissue, so you must be careful in the beginning.

"Start by lifting light weights twice a week. After four weeks you can add a third workout each week. In ten weeks, you'll start to see results."

You should, however, work with a professional trainer—and also make sure that your two or three days are not two or three consecutive days because muscles need at least 48 hours between workouts.

You have two options—free weights and weight machines, such as the Nautilus and Universal machines that are very popular at health clubs.

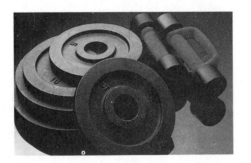

Free weights—that is, dumbbells and barbells—give you somewhat more flexibility because they don't limit your range of motion. They also improve your balance and give each muscle an equal workout.

But with a set of free weights, lifting two arms simultaneously with the same force at the same speed requires coordination and balance. It may be easier to injure yourself with free weights, although if you're paying close attention to form, you probably won't. Work with an instructor and choose which type of weights you like best.

Your muscles will thank you. You may not look like the women bodybuilders (even if you wanted to!), but you'll look good.

"Exercise will increase muscle mass even if you've been sedentary for a long time," says Dr. Simeon Margolis, professor of biological chemistry at the Johns Hopkins School of Medicine. "You begin gradually and build up. The muscles are there—they haven't gone anywhere—so you can build them up again. It's important because it takes more energy at the age of 40 than it did at 20 to maintain basic body functions and basal needs, such as heart rate and breathing. Since women over 40 are less metabolically active, they need to make more of an effort to maintain muscle and not get fleshy."

Weight lifting may make you heavier—pound for pound, muscles are denser than fat (one pound of muscle is one-half the size of fat)—but it will be a heavenly state of heaviness because your clothes will be looser. "As you exercise, you become more aware of your muscles, how they feel, what they do," explains Carol Richards Tsiames, fitness adviser and human movement specialist at the Lexington Avenue YWCA in New York City. "Muscle is heavier than fat. So you may end up weighing more but looking thinner because you will have strengthened muscles and eliminated flab."

point out that the increased supply of oxygen to the brain and the hormones that are released during exercise are natural mood elevators.

EXERCISE AND MEMORY

Exercise, specifically aerobic exercise, might improve your memory, as well. In an experiment at the U.S. Veterans Administration Hospital in Salt Lake City, Utah, a group of people averaging age 61 exercised aerobically and improved their scores significantly in six of eight tests measuring reaction time and short-term memory. Another group of like test subjects who did quick-burst workouts like pushups and light weight lifting improved in only one of the tests. The control group that did not exercise showed no memory improvement.

Research also indicates that those who exercise regularly tend to have more dominant personalities than the average person. Something about the exertion seems to shake out meekness and passivity. And a health survey conducted in Canada a few years ago revealed that "Physically active people, particularly those 45 years and over, are less likely to experience disability days or long-term activity limitation, to take drugs, or to have recently consulted a doctor. They are more likely to have a positive emotional well-being and lower blood pressure."

Don't, however, put undue pressure on yourself by chanting, with every beat of your jogging shoes as they hit the ground, "I'm going to relieve my blahs and start feeling assertive and marvelous." That's like forcing yourself to relax. Your mood will elevate only if the exercise becomes an enjoyable end in itself. Think of it as your time of day to revitalize yourself, unwind, shut out tense thoughts, and meditate while listening to your favorite music.

"You'll think of new things while you're exercising. It's great for the mind and for your creativity," says Bob Young, senior program director at the Vanderbilt YMCA in New York City.

EXERCISING FOR HEALTH
AND LONGEVITY

In our sedentary world, it's not uncommon for a person's body fat to increase by one-half a percent every year, while the lean body mass, meaning muscle and bone tissue, decreases. But there's no biological reason that aging should make this happen. Dr. Everett Smith, director of the biogerontology laboratory at the University of Wisconsin, says many people in their middle years start to use age as an excuse for inactivity. They worry about pushing their bodies too far. "Not exercising the body is like not running a car. Eventually it rusts," says Dr. Smith.

Marie Capuis, 55: Younger through Yoga

"I never exercised until I was 52. When I was 20, I had bad posture, and I could hardly bend over, but at 52, I decided I was tired of feeling tired all the time. I took up yoga. At first I could only bend a little from my waist, but I kept going to class, and now I can touch my knees with my head! And I have a vitality I've never had before. It's funny, just when I had settled my mind into the idea of getting older, I started taking the yoga classes, and I started getting younger. I do yoga for 40 minutes, six mornings a week, and twice a week I do Zen meditation with an instructor. I feel younger physically and emotionally than I ever have in my life!"

If you let things go, aging can take a toll on the body. According to Dr. Herbert A. DeVries, director of the exercise/fitness laboratory at the Andrus Gerontology Center at the University of Southern California, the maximum cardiac output, meaning the ability of the heart to pump blood, declines approximately 8 percent per decade once we reach adulthood. Blood pressure tends to rise and coronary arteries to clog with fatty deposits as we get older. The chest wall starts to stiffen, so that breathing requires more muscular effort, and we inhale less oxygen to transport to our body's multitude of cells. Skeletal muscle gradually loses strength and endurance, and 3 to 5 percent of our total muscle tissue disappears with every decade. Of course, we are losing bone mass all the time.

Before you head for the rest home, consider this fact: You can reverse much of the aging process by exercising that heart and circulatory system and those muscles and bones, and by getting that oxygen pumping into your lungs again!

Exercise has never conclusively been shown to prolong life. But, according to experts like Dr. Raymond Harris, president of the Center for the Study of Aging in Albany, New York, exercise can retard some of the functional declines that come with aging, such as the loss of muscle mass, the capacity for physical effort, flexibility, endurance, bone strength, and the efficiency of the heart and lungs. It can also help to normalize blood pressure, blood sugar, and blood cholesterol, not to mention the obvious positive effects it can have on your emotional health.

PREVENTING WEAK BONES AND PAINFUL JOINTS

Though it's important for men to exercise, it's probably even more important for women, especially those of us who are over 40, because we're more prone to overweight and osteoporosis. After menopause women can lose bone mass at a rate of about 5 percent per year. Osteoporosis is more common in older women than is rheumatoid arthritis, diabetes, heart attacks, stroke, or breast cancer—yet exercise can help ward it off, like a magic charm. In fact, exercise is so important that your gynecologist should review your exercise habits and calcium intake in addition to giving you a routine pelvic exam and Pap smear. Bone is living tissue, and as you put stress on it, it gets stronger and thicker. Women track and field athletes have bones that are about 30 percent denser than the average woman's.

Once upon a time I suppose a "Lady" might have created a scandal by running and sweating in public, but, of course, all that has changed. I remember the fragile, stooped octogenarian woman who eyed me curiously one morning when I was jogging and said, "Do ladies run, too?" Her spine showed the unmistakable effects of osteoporosis, and I wished that I could have granted her a new chance at a liberated life in this fitness-conscious era. Yet statistics today show that at least 16 million Americans over the age of 35 are physically inactive. Inactive people have a coronary death rate nearly double that of those who are active.

Coronary heart disease is still the leading cause of death in postmenopausal women, at about 260 deaths per 100,000 women per year. But exercise has been found to lower the risk. Studies also show that exercise acts to increase one's levels of high-density lipoproteins (HDL), the good fats that help protect against heart disease.

Physicians are also starting to prescribe exercise for arthritis. A dear friend who suffers from arthritis is at last convinced—thanks to my ceaseless prodding and nagging—that the best thing she can do for herself is to start a gradual exercise program. Because arthritis is so painful, many of the 40 million Americans who suffer from arthritis stop trying to move their aching joints. Unfortunately, this aggravates the problem and can lead to permanent crippling. If you have arthritis, it will really benefit you to see a physical therapist or physiatrist (medical doctor specializing in movement), who can explain how to warm up your muscles and minimize the fatigue and pain so that you get all the exercise benefits to your joints. Isometric exercises are especially good for arthritis. In such exercises muscles are alternately contracted and relaxed without any real movement, as in tensing and relaxing the buttocks muscles, or repeatedly pressing the hands together.

"If you have problems with joints, whether your problem is arthritis or not, it's better to stay away from exaggerated weight-bearing exercises like jogging. Swim instead," recommends Dr. Letha Hunter, a sports medicine specialist at the Peachtree Orthopedic Clinic in Atlanta.

THE PRE-EXERCISE PHYSICAL EXAM

Anyone over the age of 40 should have a thorough physical examination before embarking on a new exercise program. You should also have an examination of your cardiovascular system, blood pressure, muscles, and joints. Your blood should be analyzed for cholesterol and triglycerides, and you should have a resting electrocardiogram.

The examination should also include an exercise stress test. This is usually done on a stationary bicycle or a motor-powered treadmill. While you work out, the physician monitors your heartbeat, electrocardiogram, blood pressure, and sometimes the amount of oxygen you consume. The test will check out your responses to exercise and may turn up evidence of impaired heart function before you begin a strenuous program. But even if you do register some weakness of the heart, it doesn't mean you shouldn't exercise. It just means you should start more slowly, following a prescribed program that will help your heart.

Never let weakness and fatigue stand in the way of your seeing a doctor and starting an exercise program. Many people end their day exhausted, figuring they must be getting too old or working too hard, when actually the problem is that *they're not working enough*. If you push your body harder, you'll increase your lung capacity and give yourself a slower resting pulse rate so that your circulatory system doesn't have to work as hard just to make it through the day. The result: *more energy*. And you'll be truly at your peak, according to the World Health Organization's definition of health, which is "physical, mental, and social well-being, not merely the absence of disease and infirmity."

GETTING STARTED

Getting started is the hardest part of exercising. I started because a friend, Jeanne, challenged me to, and because I got tired of feeling run-down all the time. Find your own reason for motivation. If you don't have a reason that is strong enough to carry you through on your own, I suggest you take a class. Getting a buddy to exercise with you is also good for motivation. Join a health club—a small exercise studio or the Y. Feedback and praise and a pleasant social situation are helpful in inspiring you to keep going, even when you think you can't make it. Whatever sort of class you join, make sure it's close to your home or office; if it's not, you'll give up because of the inconvenience of getting there. The Y I belong to is near my apartment, but on the days when I don't have time to go there, I exercise at home with my weights while watching an early-morning talk show. And I ride an exercycle I recently bought. I also walk 25 city blocks to work, and sometimes home.

Once you become really committed to an exercise program, you'll find that it gives you energy to be more productive in other areas of your life. You'll start looking for excuses to exercise and start thinking of ways to overcome the inconveniences, just because it makes life so much more enjoyable. If the weather is bad, I exercise indoors. If it's going to be a crowded day, and mine often are, I get up an hour earlier to exercise. One of my friends is blessed with a particularly cooperative family, and she's been known to get children, nieces, nephews, and great-aunts to join her on family hikes. And once you cross that threshold from some-time exerciser to fitness enthusiast, you'll never let lethargy or emotional stress keep you from it—because exercise will become your escape from tension and worry.

If you do get so busy that you miss a few days, don't waste effort in chastising yourself. Just pick up where you left off. Make the most of the days you *do* exercise; don't put yourself down for those you don't.

START SLOWLY

You may wonder about injuries. As I said previously, you should see your doctor before you begin exercising, and it's a good idea to work with an exercise instructor and approach exercise slowly.

You might begin by running for 5, 10, or 15 minutes at a time, three times a week; then gradually work up to more. Don't *ever* run without warming up and warming down, including stretching exercises. Run on level ground and, if possible, on grass or a track that's made for runners. You might want to opt for an aerobic dance class, which will provide a level, carpeted floor and a trained instructor who will guide you through proper warm-ups and cool-downs and show you which part of the foot to land on so that your joints don't take an unnecessary beating.

WHAT TO WEAR

When you run or take an aerobics class, wear shorts or a sweatsuit, depending on the weather. Sweatsuits are better than leotards, which tend to bind. The new Gore-Tex running suits are lightweight and keep you warm in winter—they are certainly worth trying. Never wear those expensive synthetic garments that sport shops bill as "sauna suits," designed to make you sweat so that you ostensibly shed extra pounds. Actually, they only make you lose water and that gives you the illusion of losing weight; however, that water loss is hazardous to your health.

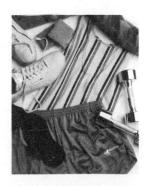

Warming-Up, Cooling-Down, and Checking Your Pulse

Before you start an aerobic workout, warm up with a few light stretching exercises (but not "bounce" stretching), and begin to run, bicycle, walk, swim, or whatever your method may be, slowly, for a five- to ten-minute warm-up. Gradually begin to pick up the momentum. Monitor yourself the first time after ten minutes by checking your pulse to see if you're getting a proper workout. Do not stop moving while you check your pulse. This will show you how your heart is performing. Once you've started exercising regularly, you should check your pulse at the end of each aerobic workout, just before the cool-down.

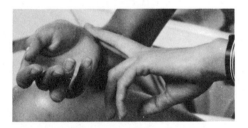

This is how you check your pulse: Lightly press two fingers against one of the pulse points: the radial artery on the thumb side of the wrist, the temporal artery in front of and slightly above the ear, the carotid artery on the neck about halfway between the sternal notch and the earlobe, or the left chest just beneath the breast. Though each person differs, doctors and physical educators use the following formula to determine what your pulse should be as you exercise: Subtract your age from 220, then multiply by 0.75. If you're 40, your exercise pulse rate should be in the range of 135, but you'll see from the table that your actual target zone can be anywhere from 128 to 155 beats per minute. Don't count your pulse for an entire minute, however, because it will begin to slow down very quickly, and you won't get an accurate picture of the way your heart is working while you exercise. Find the beat, count it for ten seconds, then multiply the number of beats by six. Then check the table, and see if you're really getting a proper workout. If your heart rate falls in the 70 percent level below the target range and you are in good shape, it means you should be exercising more vigorously. If it is in the 85 percent level, this means you're working your heart too hard, and you should slow down.

After the workout, ease yourself back into a relaxed state with a five- to ten-minute cool-down. Don't skip this; an abrupt halt may trap all the blood in the muscles that have suddenly stopped moving. Then the circulation to your brain, heart, or intes-

WATER PLEASE

That brings up the question of how to eat and drink to accommodate your newly active life. Drink water! And drink some more—it's the best thing for your body. It will guard against dehydration, so drink up before you start working out. After the workout drink until your thirst is totally quenched, and if you exercise for more than 45 minutes, have a few sips of water between takes. Drink plain, pure water. Drink bottled

tine can slow down and produce dizziness or faintness, palpitating heartbeats, or nausea. Do a series of exercises and stretches similar to those in the warm-up, but take it more slowly this time. Stretch slowly, languorously, decreasing the speed of your movements until finally, you're not moving at all.

Maximal Attainable Heart Rate and Target Zone

This table shows that as we grow older, the highest heart rate that can be reached during all-out effort falls. These numerical values are "average" values for age. Note that one-third of the population may differ from these values. It is quite possible that a normal 50-year-old man may have a maximum heart rate of 195 or that a 30-year-old man might have a maximum of only 168. The same limitations apply to the 70 percent and 85 percent of maximum lines.

mineral water if you like, but don't waste your money on those soft drinks billed as "super thirst quenchers." They're full of sugar and salt and not nearly so effective as water. And those commercials showing superstar athletes refreshing themselves after the game with major name-brand soft drinks, especially colas, should have us all picketing the agencies that dream up those ads.

NUTRITION FOR EXERCISE

You've probably heard about carbohydrate loading for athletes. Complex carbohydrates (pastas, whole grain cereals and breads, rice, and potatoes, for example) are essential to your muscle endurance. If they're the mainstay of your diet, you'll never have to worry about "loading" them—your muscles will just function at optimal strength, thanks to your sensible combination of diet and exercise.

It's hard to exercise first thing in the morning with your blood sugar feeling sluggish, so you may want to have a glass of fruit juice, as I do, before you start. Don't, however, exercise on a full stomach. You'll know you've made a mistake by the immediate indigestion. Loading up on carbohydrates in the last hour before exercising will impose too much demand on your muscle's glycogen deposits—distracting the muscles from the job of exercising. Your muscles also need some extra nutrients when you're exercising.

Active women most commonly need extra B_2 (riboflavin) and iron. Try a daily multivitamin and mineral supplement, with about 100 percent of the Recommended Dietary Allowance (RDA) of each nutrient, as your body's insurance.

FINDING YOUR FAVORITE EXERCISE

"You can reverse the aging process and tone the most neglected body with aerobic exercise," says Dr. Hunter. If you can't jog because of weak feet, ankles, knees, or other problems, you can race-walk. If that bores you, you can swim or do dance exercises. If done for at least 20 minutes at a time, all of these exercises will work the cardiovascular system, will tone muscles, and prevent and restore bone loss. (Note: Swimming is less successful in restoring bone loss than the weight-bearing exercises. Swimming is a perfect exercise in every sense but this.)

You have to be patient. Exercise does work, but it takes more than a few casual attempts. "You can shape up at any age," says Dr. Hunter. "You may not see instantaneous results, but you will get results. It will help you through menopause because it benefits you psychologically. Also, if you look better—and with exercise you will look better—you will feel better."

If you decide to start by running, you must advance slowly. "You don't become a marathon runner overnight," cautions Dr. Hunter. "You must also have proper warm-up and cool-down exercises, before and after running, and the proper shoes. It's best to run on a track with a dirt surface, or on asphalt, both of which are more shock-absorbent than city concrete.

Running is the most visible form of exercise these days. But if that's not for you, there are other exercise programs you can start.

I did say you should see your physician before you begin exercising, but don't drive there—walk! I can't think of a better way to start the momentum, enjoy the fresh air, and start exercising your heart and lungs than to employ the exercise you've been doing all your life, but which you may have come to neglect a bit in our motorized age.

WALKING

A brisk four-mile walk for an hour every other day will decrease body fat, increase the strength and endurance of your leg muscles, relieve stress and anxiety, and give you a good aerobic workout in the bargain. You need no special skills or coordination, no special gear except for a comfortable pair of walking shoes. (Check out a sporting goods shop for a good, sturdy pair.)

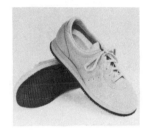

Start by walking one mile at a time. When you go to the sporting goods shop for your shoes, you might also want to pick up a pedometer, which you can carry along on each jaunt to get a fair idea of how far you've walked; gradually work up to four miles within an hour. I promise that from this one pleasant hour of brisk movement, you'll find a new joy in living. Yes, an hour.

I know, it's easy enough to feel all inspired and motivated to exercise, harder to actually take the time to do it regularly. "You must structure life for an hour a day for the self and learn not to juggle too much," says Bob Young, senior program director at the Vanderbilt YMCA in New York City, the Y I visit several times a week. And start slowly—in fact, if you haven't been exercising, Young recommends exercising only every other day for the first few weeks.

"Your muscles will be sore," he says, "In fact, that's one simple way that you can measure your success—are your muscles less sore this week than they were last week? It will take 24 to 36 hours for that soreness to go away, so you must exercise only every other day at first," he says. And another way that you'll know the hard work is paying off, says Young, is on the scales. "If you burn 500 calories a day more than you take in, you will lose a pound a week."

Besides that hour to yourself—and I assure you, you'll soon begin to look forward to it—there must be somewhere else that you can walk instead of drive. How far is the supermarket, the office, even the tennis court? I realize that your friends may think you're crazy to walk, but your svelte figure will give you the last laugh. Take it from me—I've even walked in Los Angeles, where nobody walks! (You may need a smog mask there, however.)

RACE-WALKING

If you've worked up to walking at a fast clip, you can step up your pace and become a devotee of race-walking. If you don't trust your ankles, feet, or knees to hold up through a jog, or if you've tried jogging in the past and they've given you problems, race-walking is the answer. Because it's easy on the body—there's no pounding on your joints and feet—race-walking is an especially good anti-aging exercise. I race-walk sometimes when I feel the slightest twinge of pain in my legs or back from running, knowing that even on that city pavement, race-walking won't hurt. It's something to consider if you're a city dweller. Ruella Frank, a New York City psychotherapist and movement therapist, says it has all sorts of extra benefits over jogging. "You don't bounce up and down and put a great deal of stress on your joints and back. You always have one foot on the ground, so you're always in a balanced position—unlike with running, where two legs are off the ground at the same time, so that when you hit the pavement again, all your joints are stressed. Race-walking stretches and flexes your ankles. Also, it helps correct your posture. Many women over 40 start to cave in at the chest and get a rounding of the upper back. The race-walking posture, which keeps your head in a comfortably erect position, your spine aligned, and your legs doing the work, corrects that." She also says that race-walking will help to ease that tension between the shoulder blades that so many of us endure. "That kind of tension puts pressure on the nerves that go to the heart and lungs," says Frank. "By swinging your arms when you race-walk, you loosen up on that tension, as well as the tension in the back and the neck, areas that tend to stiffen as we get older.

Race-walking is strenuous exercise—as you'll find out quickly. It will leave you much too sweaty to be presentable at the office, so I'd suggest that you don't plan to do it on the way to work. (Of course, you could bring sweat clothes to work and race-walk home!) Start the program by race-walking for 15 minutes at a time, work up to 20 minutes, and eventually to an hour.

The flabless, youthful-looking, 40-year-old Ms. Frank race-walks for an hour at a time, five days a week, and swears by it. "It exercises more muscles than jogging does," she says. "About the same number of muscles get a workout as in swimming. That includes the muscles on the outside of the thigh, so it's a perfect exercise for working off saddlebags."

I also recommend *Walking—the Pleasure Exercise* by Mort Malkin (Emmaus, Pa.: Rodale Press, 1986) if you are interested in starting a walking program.

Here's how to race-walk:

✔ Start by letting your arms hang loosely and extending one leg in front of you. Take your normal gait and exaggerate it.

✔ Stretch out the heel of one foot, push off with the other leg, and walk fast. The motion is push, reach, push, reach . . . the back foot pushes while the front foot reaches. When you see professional race-walkers move, they look as though they're gliding.

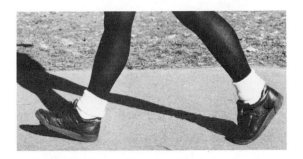

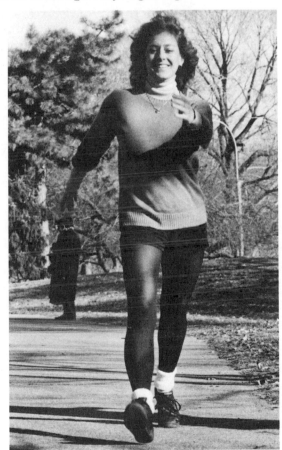

✔ Meanwhile, keep swinging your arms. Swing them much faster and wider than you do in a normal walk. (The fact is, some people don't swing their arms enough normally.) By swinging your arms, you're working your upper body.

✔ The next more advanced position is to carry your lower arms at right angles to your body and swing them on the same arc as when they were hanging. Your hands are in a comfortable fist position. Imagine that they are alternately punching an imaginary dot six inches in front of your breastbone and that your elbows are poking a cloud behind you. This will give you the correct arc of your arms.

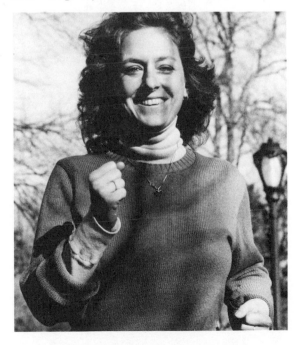

✔ When the weight is on the front foot, keep that leg straight. You want to take as long a stride as possible. One way to take a longer stride is to keep your back heel down as long as you can and keep the front leg extended as much as you can.

Images to Correct Posture

Using a body movement practice called idiokinesis, in which you conjure up special images for certain parts of your body that you want to relax and strengthen, can improve your posture. Ruella Frank, a New York City psychotherapist and movement therapist, uses idiokinesis in her practice. She suggests the following three images.

Puppet on a String Image

Balloon Image

Dinosaur Tail Image

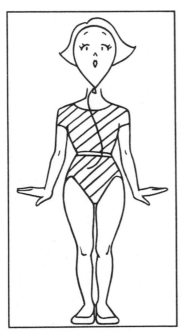

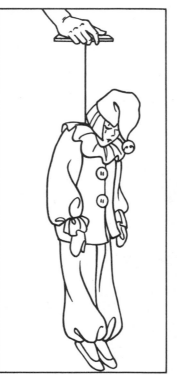

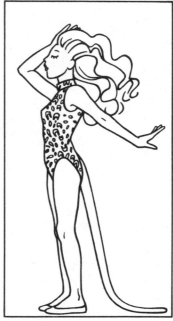

Imagine your head floating skyward like a balloon. You *just* imagine; you don't do anything special. (As you imagine, muscle tissues will start to change and transform on their own. This is the nature of the exercises.) Most of us push our heads forward to meet the world; this image allows the head to reposition appropriately.

Picture a string from your seventh cervical, which is the biggest bone at the end of the neck, and a puppeteer holding the string, pulling your neck up skyward. This will help your spine stretch and lengthen.

Visualize a tail, like a dinosaur tail, at the end of your spine, hanging down and descending into the earth. That will make your pelvis hang smoothly and will smooth out all the muscles of the buttocks.

SWIMMING

If you're lucky enough to have your own pool, you'll certainly want to use it. If you don't, you might want to find a Y or health club with a pool. Some mornings I swim for 20 minutes at the Y before work, and I go through the entire day smiling.

How do you swim for maximum aerobic benefit? Not by just paddling about or floating in the water, says cardiologist Lenore R. Zohman, M.D., in *Beyond Diet . . . Exercise Your Way to Fitness and Heart Health* (Englewood Cliffs, N. J.: CPC International, 1974), an excellent little booklet. (For a copy of this public service pamphlet, write to Mazola Oil Exercise Book, Department ZJH, Box 307, Coventry, CT 06238.) "The stroke to be used must be decided upon if cardiovascular conditioning is sought since the fitness process is accomplished more readily if one uses the same group of muscles. Try the breaststroke and check yourself by counting your heart rate after leisurely swimming for 5 minutes continuously. This is your warm-up rate. Then swim more vigorously and faster for 5 to 10 minutes to determine whether you are in your target zone. If this pace does it, your program will be to swim at that pace for 20 minutes without stopping. When you finish, stay in the water and rest for at least 5 minutes before getting out. The water pressure will help your circulation to adjust after the strenuous effort. It is not necessary to cool down in the usual sense after swimming, since body temperature, which ordinarily rises with exercise, has been prevented from rising by the coolness of the water."

A noontime swim is my favorite quick break when I can sneak off to the Y in the middle of a hectic day. Oh, I know, you have to dry your hair afterward and reapply makeup and all that, but even if I don't have time for a cosmetic touchup after swimming, the glow in my skin and eyes and the rejuvenated feeling I have all over more than compensates for a little hair out of place. I go back to the office and people say, "What happened to you, Donna? You left the office looking haggard, and now you're back looking terrific."

ROPE SKIPPING AND ROPE JUMPING

By doing rope skipping (one foot always on the ground) and rope jumping (both feet off the ground at once), you can vary your workout so that you do both, and you can run in place as well. Because rope skipping and rope jumping are such intense exercises, you should begin gradually to avoid speeding up your heart rate too fast.

"First make sure the rope is the right length—both ends should reach up to the armpits when the center of the rope's length is held under your feet. Then work into a sensible program," says Dr. Zohman

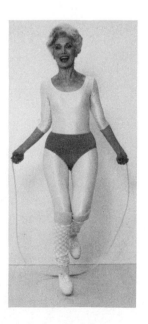

in her pamphlet. She cites authority Dr. Kaare Rodahl, who has devised a plan for jumping rope. Here's how you go about it:

✔ First week: Warm up by jumping in place without the rope 100 times. Next, skip rope 50 times at a comfortable speed. Increase 10 skips a day for the remaining four sessions in that "week" (a week is defined as five exercising days). At the end of the week, you will reach 90 skips.

✔ Second week: Warm up with 50 hops. Then do 100 skips, adding 10 skips per day until you are doing 140 skips at the end of the week.

✔ Third week: Warm up with 50 hops. Then do 100 skips. Rest for 15 to 30 seconds. Repeat 100 skips.

✔ Fourth week and thereafter: Continue to add skips to the point of breathlessness. Your ultimate aim is to reach 500 skips in five minutes.

BICYCLING

Once you're in shape for it, there's nothing more pleasurable than a long Saturday afternoon bicycle ride. Unlike other exercise programs, this is one that can actually get you somewhere. If I didn't live in a traffic-ridden Manhattan (and have a tendency, as my husband says, "to space out on the sights and forget where I am"), I might bicycle to work. Even here when the transit workers went on strike a number of years ago, bicycling became a popular mode of transportation. If you're not a space cadet, like I am, try buying a bicycle and leaving your car in the garage more often—you'll get where you're going and get all the benefits of aerobic exercise, too.

Whether you're cycling to get somewhere, riding on a bicycle path, or using a stationary bike for a workout, your guiding principles are the same as for any other exercise regimen. Use a warm-up-stimulus-cool-down pattern with 20 minutes as your target range at least three non-consecutive days of cycling a week, says Dr. Zohman in her book. She goes on to say:

When using a *rolling bicycle,* you may increase the intensity of your efforts by pedaling faster, or pedaling over hilly terrain, or using the higher gears on your bicycle. Try to plan your route, for example, so you ride over a flat stretch for 5 to 10 minutes, then up and down some hills for 20 minutes, then back to the flat for the cool-down. Or ride with lower gears, making it easier during warm-up and cool-down, and use mostly your own effort rather than mechanical advantage during the stimulus period. If the entire bicycle path is flat, ride very rapidly during stimulus as compared to warm-up and cool-down. From your pulse rate responses you can decide whether your program is adequate . . . .

In using a *stationary bicycle* or bicycle ergometer, it is important to adjust the seat height and the handgrips correctly. If the seat is too low or too high, the leg muscles will not be able to function the most efficiently and much energy will be wasted struggling against the bicycle. With your toes on the pedal, there should be a small bend at the knee when the pedal is in the fully down position.

The exercise challenge on the stationary bicycle is not provided by hills, speed, or gears, but rather by the resistance knob. The expensive indoor models (bicycle ergometers) cost more money because the mechanism for introducing resistance to pedaling is reliable and reproducible. If a certain amount of resistance is applied at a particular setting on one day, that setting will give the exact same resistance the next. The less expensive cycle exercisers may have a knob that applies resistance, but there are rarely any gradations on this knob. Even if there were such gradations or settings, the amount of resistance applied to pedaling during one session might differ from that at the same setting during the next because it is a less precise exercise instrument.

Initially begin at the number 1 for your warm-up, and try setting 2 for a stimulus period setting. Take your pulse rate after five minutes at each level to determine whether you are on target, and adjust the number of turns of the knob to give you the proper heart rate. Your pedaling rate should remain constant at either 50 or 60 revolutions per minute. That is, your right foot should move toward the floor 50 or 60 times each minute. An ordinary music metronome will be very helpful in keeping the rate constant. Realize that the number of turns may be somewhat different from day to day—but not that different—and that your heart rate response, not the resistance setting, is the ultimate guideline even on the most expensive bike.

STRETCHING EXERCISES

While aerobic exercise is the ultimate anti-aging secret and the *only* way to keep your heart, lungs, and bones in shape, stretching exercises are also important for conditioning your body, improving your aerobic performance, and guarding against injuries. If you follow the Pilates technique (many exercise studios do—ask around) or buy the book *The Pilates Method of Physical and Mental Conditioning* (New York: Doubleday & Company, 1980) by Philip Friedman and Gail Eisen, you can get a complete stretching and even some aerobic workout. Personally, I like to make the Pilates exercises a supplement to my aerobic routine. I do stretch exercises three days a week and do something aerobic three alternating days.

Women in their fifties have actually increased their mobility by four inches using the Pilates stretches. The exercises begin with your lying on the floor doing abdominal stretching exercises, and then limbering the hamstrings, Achilles tendons, and other tight areas. Next, you advance to a sitting position, then a standing one, in a gradual process of stretching and strengthening.

Romana Kryzanowska, the director of the Isotoner Fitness Center, a Pilates exercise facility in New York City—in fact, it's New York's oldest health club, having been around since 1923—is a walking testament to the technique she teaches. Though she is a grandmother, she is the very picture of radiance and vitality. At this world-renowned studio, she works with clients whose ages range from their teens right up into their eighties.

"You can improve flexibility at any age," says Romana. But you'll hardly know that you're working so many muscles when you start this technique. Pilates aims to never leave you sore.

"After the first session, a client may feel like we haven't done anything," says Romana. "But that's the way we want them to feel. Ninety percent of our exercise is done lying down. You can even do aerobic exercises with your back flat on a surface. You don't have to jump up and down; you can lie flat and flap your arms, as in the first move we do, the Hundred." (We show you how to do the Hundred on the opposite page.)

Romana says, "Our major effort is put into strengthening the abdominal band—this is the powerhouse of the body. If this is kept strong, the rest of the body will be flexible and move freely and easily. One of the primary aims of our exercises is to create long, thin, strengthened muscles.

"One of my clients came to me with arthritis, a bad back, and diabetes. She could only work ten minutes before she was exhausted. After a few months she could work an hour; she feels wonderful."

Romana has inspired me—and if I ever feel so draggy that I can hardly lift a hand, I visit her studio and am reminded of how many people have been practically reborn just by exercising.

THE PILATES METHOD: THE HUNDRED

If you do nothing else, I urge you to try the Pilates Hundred as shown here—I think it will inspire you to get going, too. It stimulates your circulation and breathing—in fact, part of the exercise is an aerobic one that you do flat on your back!

✔ Begin by anchoring yourself. Lie on your back on a mat with your arms at your sides, palms down. Anchor yourself in place by pressing your spine to the mat. Try to make your navel touch your spine, but don't suck your stomach in or hold your breath. Imagine, instead, a heavy weight pressing down your middle.

✔ Bend your knees and bring them to your chest, pressing your spine closer to the mat.

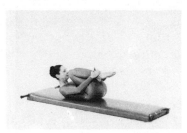

✔ Straighten your legs, keeping them together, to about a right angle with the floor. Keep your chin on your chest. Hold your legs straight, and toes pointed.

✔ Now lower your legs until your spine begins to arch off the mat. *Stop.* Press your spine down, raising your legs slightly if you need to keep your spine on the floor. [Editor's Note: Straight leg exercises can create problems for those who have back problems, particularly the lower back. If you are one

of these, or if you have any back weakness at all, it would be wise to skip this step in the method.]

✔ Lift your hands off the mat, about six inches, and hold them next to your body, palms down, with your arms and wrists straight, reaching away from your shoulders with your fingertips, as illustrated by model Nancy Zeckendorf.

✔ Now for the actual movement. Pump your arms up and down rapidly a few inches, moving them toward the ceiling and then toward the mat, in short, vigorous strokes, for

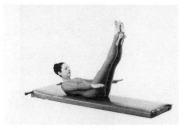

5 counts. Do this 4 times—20 strokes in all. Work up gradually to 100 pumping motions (hence, the name) by adding 5 at a time.

✔ Breathe in for 5 pumping motions, then out for the next 5. Thus, if you do 100, you'll take 10 deep breaths altogether. Empty your lungs competely with each breath.

The form is very important, even if your body feels stiff at first. If your neck muscles get tired, lower your head to the mat for a few pumping motions, then raise it again if you can. If your legs start to sink as you move, raise them a little higher. Eventually, your toes should be on a line with your eyes. If you can't reach that position at first, just lower your legs as far as you can while keeping your spine pressed flat to the mat. And keep your eyes on your stomach—make sure it doesn't budge.

THE PILATES METHOD: THE CIRCLE STRETCH— A GREAT EXERCISE TO DO AT THE OFFICE

If you're desk-bound most of the day and you find that you get stiff from sitting, Pilates has some stretch exercises that you can do on the job, too. Lift yourself from that chair, stand beside the wall, and try the Circle Stretch. Here's how:

✔ Lean against the wall with your arms straight in front of you. Position your heels as close to the wall as possible. At the same time, keep your back flat against the wall and your feet together. (Each time you do this exercise, move your feet a little closer to the wall until eventually, they touch the wall.) Keep your stomach held in.

✔ Now, lift your arms forward in front of you, up to the wall behind you, and then down to the side slowly, as if you were making large arm circles. Breathe in deeply while raising your arms slowly, and breathe out deeply as you lower them. Do this three times, then reverse directions. Now you can go back to your desk refreshed.

Just try a few simple exercises if you're not quite ready to take on swimming or track. Even a little exercise is going to make you start to want more—and then, I guarantee, you're going to feel great once you get started. Over-40s women, keep it up, and we can take over the world. There are going to be enough of us to do it, so why not now?

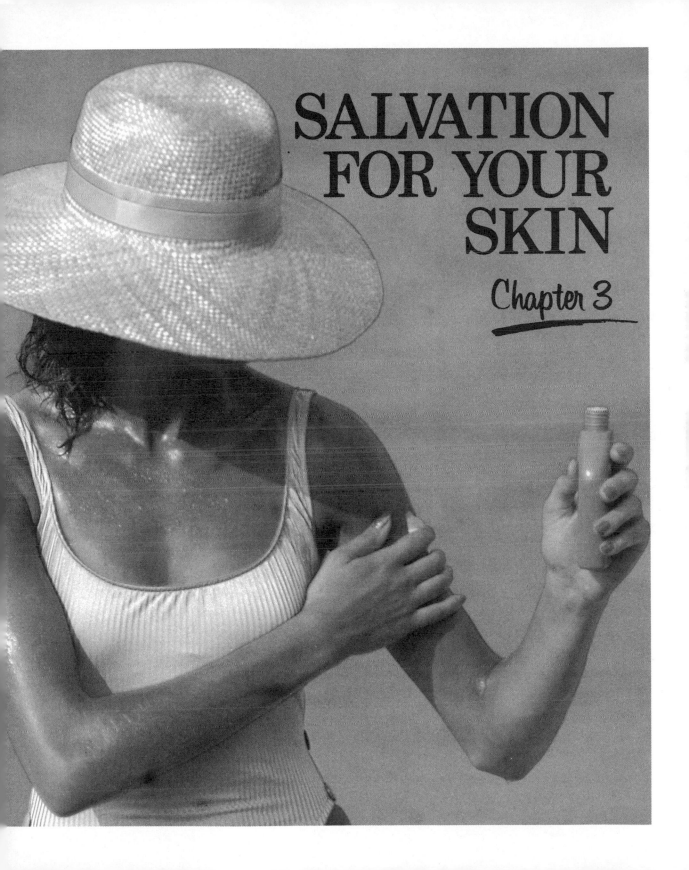

SALVATION FOR YOUR SKIN

Chapter 3

True, we've earned every line we've got. No one wants a face that's a blank page. But, at the same time, the sags and bags and little furrowed waves gathering around the cheeks can be a depressing sight to even the most sanguine among us.

So, now that we're 40 plus we ask, "Can anything be done?"

Of course. The first thing you can do is get a better understanding of your skin's natural friends and enemies. Certain things will contribute to the health and vitality of skin, while others will dehydrate it and age it prematurely.

Now that I'm 48, my skin is drier, so I use superfatted soap and Lubriderm lotion. If I keep my diet as salt-free as possible, the areas under my eyes are noticeably less puffy, and when they become puffy, I put wet tea bags on them.

About a year ago, my hands were getting dry and my nails were chipping. A manicurist told me to switch from my generic brand of dishwashing detergent to Ivory. I did. This is an unpaid endorsement. My nails grew stronger; my hands were softer.

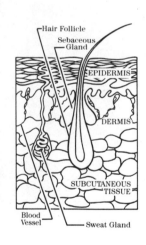

Hair Follicle
Sebaceous Gland
EPIDERMIS
DERMIS
SUBCUTANEOUS TISSUE
Blood Vessel
Sweat Gland

YOUR SKIN: WHAT'S IT ALL ABOUT?

Such measures are certainly worthwhile, and I encourage you to seek out every helpful hint you can get. But if you want to understand good skin care and make sense out of the many new products on the market with pseudo-technical names and claims, you need to know what your skin is really all about—exactly what it is and how it functions.

The outer layer of skin is the epidermis, which in itself is four layers. The outermost layer, the one that you can actually see, is the stratum corneum, made up of flat, dry skin cells. Beneath the epidermis is the dermis, the thickest layer. The dermis is your skin's support system. It is made up largely of collagen and elastin (the sun's favorite targets), substances that make your skin smooth, durable, and resilient. Without them, you wouldn't be able to flex your face—smile, talk, or eat—and know that your skin would return to its original position.

The innermost layer of the epidermis, commonly called the basal layer, is the font of your skin's new cells. Here, new cells are born constantly, and they are born healthy, fresh, and plump. However, they must journey through layer upon layer of the epidermis to reach the outer layer, and by the time they arrive, they are rarely in the same condition as when they started. For the outer layer is always shedding off its dead cells; in fact, the whole layer regenerates itself every 28 to 30 days.

The blood vessels in the dermis are there to deliver oxygen to the basal layers of your epidermis. When these capillaries break, often due to sun damage, the blood spreads into the tissue, creating discolorations in the skin. And spider veins, those blotchy, little, red, weblike marks are merely the evidence of the capillary network underneath. People with delicate, translucent skin are much more prone to revealing spider veins and broken capillaries than are people with darker complexions. If this applies to you, your best defense is to limit your exposure to the sun, or to get very familiar with zinc oxide, the thick white stuff I apply and reapply to my nose.

(If you have spider veins—or broken capillaries—a dermatologist can treat them easily and painlessly. Electrodesiccation, or "drying up" of the affected area, can be done right in the doctor's office and rarely leaves any visible traces.)

THE BASICS OF SKIN CARE: CLEANSING—FIRST THINGS FIRST

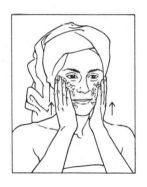

As we grow older, it becomes increasingly important to handle our skin with care because its ability to withstand irritation diminishes every year. With age, skin begins to thin out, and the natural production of oils slows down. That's why our skin feels drier and more sensitive than it did in our salad days. So the way we cleanse our skin really counts; improper washing and the use of harsh soaps can be harmful.

Obviously, we've all been washing our faces long enough to make it almost second nature, but many women don't realize that how they wash can make an enormous difference. The temperature of the water should be tepid, *never* scalding and *never* ice cold. You should gently work up a lather, using slow upward motions on your face. Take care not to pull your skin downward, particularly in the fragile areas around your eyes. This only accentuates any sagging or looseness in the skin. *Do not rub your skin.* Then rinse it thoroughly with water and gently pat it dry with a soft, cotton towel. Harsh, abrasive washcloths and towels tug at your skin.

Depending on your skin type, the accompanying guide should help you to decide which soap or cleanser is best for you. I've included oily skin although it is uncommon after age 40. My skin, which once was oily, has turned decidedly dry over the last five years.

The Best Cleansing Agents for Your Type of Skin

Generally, the categories of skin are broken up into normal, dry, and oily; the rate of secretion of sebum, the skin's own natural oil, determines which type yours is. Sebum gives skin its softness, moistness, and glow. Sebum forms an acid mantle on the skin's surface that protects it against external drying influences and bacteria.

✔ **Normal skin** produces the correct amount of sebum and has enough cellular water retention to ensure its own natural moistness. Keeping this skin type clean is necessary to remove not only dirt but also the pileup of cells that daily rise to the skin's surface and die. These cells must be removed to make room for new ones; otherwise the skin becomes dull and the pores become clogged, so that the sebum isn't able to reach the surface.

Clean normal skin with a mild cleanser that can be rinsed off easily with plain water.

✔ **Dry skin** has barely visible pores, but it wrinkles faster than other types. The problem is a slow production of sebum, resulting in a lack of the protective acid mantle on the skin's surface. This is generally due to an improper functioning of the sebaceous glands. Another cause of dryness is a lack of water in the deeper cellular layers of the skin. These conditions can be inherited, or they can be the result of poor health. Also, as we get older, these protective processes slow down.

External influences that dry the skin's surface are harsh weather, central heating, and the overuse of strong alkali soaps and dehydrating alcohol-based astringents. The balance of water retention in the skin's cells can be affected by incautious dieting, which often goes hand in hand with decreased water intake.

The skin's balance can change, making a normal or even an oily type of skin dry. Wrinkles are more likely to embed themselves in dry skin, and moistness also keeps dry skin from flaking and becoming rough and irritated. So for many rea-

sons it's necessary to keep this type of skin moist. Therefore, watch your diet, drink enough water, and avoid the dehydrating influence of alcoholic beverages. Avoid overexposure to the sun and other harsh weather conditions, or at least wear sunscreens to protect your skin against them.

Strong soaps and astringents should be avoided, although an occasional soaping with a mild castile soap or an application of a gentle lotion can't hurt the skin. In general, oil-based cleansers, lotions, masks, and saunas should be used on dry skin. Moisturizers need to be applied constantly to the skin's surface to make up for its lack of an acid mantle.

✔ **Oily skin,** seldom a problem of women over 40, produces too much sebum, giving it a shiny, large-pored, often sallow appearance. Overproduction of the sebaceous glands is the result of endocrine imbalance. Oily skin can also be part of your inherited chemical makeup. Many women go through life with oily skin, and they're in luck in this area: Even late in life they are less likely to wrinkle. Wrinkles don't linger in well-lubricated skins.

On the other hand, oily skins are more likely to be victim to blackheads, pimples, and coarse pores. This is due to clogged pores, resulting from a mixture of external dirt and pollution secretion. Cleanliness is extremely important to oily skins to remove excess pore-clogging oils and the dead cells that cause the complexion to appear sallow.

Oily skin should not be cleaned with heavy creams since they block pores. A mild castile soap makes a good cleanser.

MOISTURE: YOUR SKIN CAN'T LIVE WITHOUT IT

One of the telltale signs of aging skin is that it begins to lose its ability to retain moisture. Yet moisture is absolutely vital for keeping skin soft, supple, and strokable. Without it, skin is rough, cracked, and scaly. And nature works against you in many ways: the sun, wind, and cold all rob your skin of its precious moisture. When the relative humidity becomes lower than about 25 percent—in desert conditions, airplane cabins, and even in heated rooms during the winter, your skin needs an extra heavy dose of moisturizer. If your home or apartment is especially dry in winter, buy a humidifier and let it battle central heating. My English friend, Eva, says that women in her country credit their lovely skin to the common lack of central heating. Plants, lots of them all around the house, also build the moisture in your environment. Your skin can also use an extra dose of moisturizing lotion.

A moisturizer works something like a protective shield, allowing the outer layer to build up natural moisture and keep the skin cells hydrated. The basis of a moisturizer is its emollient, or oil, which works to lock moisture in. And the most effective emollients are the simplest ones: petroleum jelly, mineral oil, lanolin, and cocoa butter.

The best way to use a moisturizer is to apply it when your skin is *already slightly damp*, because the skin cells are retaining water. And different parts of your body need varying amounts of moisture. For example, the especially delicate area around the eyes often calls for more moisturizing, while the area around the nose may be much less dry.

Don't be deceived by fancy merchandising and astronomical prices. If you are so inclined, you can easily spend a small fortune on moisturizers alone. I use Lubriderm, a lightweight lotion that costs $3.97 for a bottle at my local discount drugstore. Pond's and Nivea products are also good. And, I also use petroleum jelly. "Vaseline is the best, the number-one moisturizer," says Dr. Albert Kligman, a professor of dermatology at the University of Pennsylvania School of Medicine and director of the school's Clinic for Aging Skin. "Lanolin is good, too. Money has nothing to do with it. You buy glamour, fragrance, and the way it goes on. A more expensive moisturizer may be nicer, but it won't be more effective. The oilier a moisturizer, the better."

Many cosmetics companies make fantastic promises on behalf of their moisturizers—rejuvenation, renewal, radiance, you name it. The ingredients they include often sound very seductive, but their claims are generally unsubstantiated. For example, collagen and elastin, the two proteins that give your skin its support and firmness, are often listed on the label. When added to a moisturizer, however, these won't firm up your skin as part of a topical application.

Homemade Moisturizers

Glycerin and Honey Moisturizer

Mix 9 parts of glycerin with 1 part honey. Blend thoroughly. Smooth this all over the face, including the area around the eyes. Keep it on all day if you can, and wear it overnight.

Cucumber Moisturizer

Keep half a peeled, crisp cucumber in the refrigerator to use as a skin moisturizer. Rub it all over your face and feel its cooling and moisturizing effects, particularly soothing to irritated skin. Cleopatra was supposed to have used this simple remedy, and our own history tells us that pioneer women used to cut open a cucumber at the end of a day in the fields and rub it on to freshen their sun-parched skins.

Lettuce Leaf Moisturizer

Simmer lettuce leaves for a couple of hours in enough distilled water to keep them from scorching in the pan. Cool and apply the liquid lightly to the face as is or mix with yogurt. Leave it on to soothe as long as is convenient. The French peasants have long used moisturizing lettuce juice to soothe angry, irritated skin.

FACIALS, MASKS, AND BATHS

There are easily a thousand ways to pamper your skin. Since the beginning of time, women have been experimenting with clay, mud, salts, oils, and herbs, trying to come up with the perfect anti-aging recipe. I'm sorry to say that the perfect one hasn't been found. I do know, though, from much experience concocting, testing, and evaluating, that there are truly beneficial treatments that are fun to try, easy to incorporate into a skin-care regimen. These treatments will, at least in part, make your skin feel like it does when you come out of a fancy New York City facial salon.

A facial mask is spread on the face, allowed to dry, and then peeled off or rinsed off with warm water. It removes dead cells from the skin's surface (this is called exfoliation) and temporarily tightens the skin. Like a mask, a bath can be therapeutic, physically and psychologically, too. Soaking in a warm (never scalding) bath can revitalize a tired body, a worn-out spirit, and help rid you of "winter itch."

One word of caution about masks and facials. In order to remove the dead skin cells, you need to be sure that they will be peeled off gently. Any mask that does this act of sloughing off, or exfoliating, by abrading your skin is too harsh. Avoid any mask with abrasive particles or so-called cleansing grains. They can wreak havoc on older skin. Here are some of my favorite masks:

Avocado Mask

Mash a ripe avocado with some vegetable oil until the mixture is as creamy as possible. Rub it into your skin, and let it remain there for 10 to 15 minutes. Rinse with warm water, and behold the smooth glow!

Banana Mask

Mash a ripe banana until it is a smooth paste, and rub it into your face. Rinse off after 15 to 20 minutes. Natural banana oils will penetrate the skin, relieving dryness.

Olive Oil Mask

Soak cotton pads with warm olive oil. Have a hot towel ready. Cover your face with the pads, and place the towel over them. Leave on until the towel becomes cool. Repeat if necessary, but don't wash off.

Tomato or Papaya Mask

Slice a ripe tomato as thinly as possible. Apply the slices to your face, and leave on for 10 to 15 minutes. Use a slice to rub the juices into your skin after the treatment. The tomato works like a face peel (or exfoliant) to remove all the dead skin from the surface, leaving your face glossy and smooth. You can accomplish the same exfoliate action with papaya. I know you'd rather eat a papaya, but it works beautifully to remove dry, dead skin from your entire body. Just stand in the tub and rub it all over you. Let it soak in, then take a soft cloth or your hand and rub your skin, watching dry flakes rub off. Don't let anyone watch you do this, however, or they'll think you're mad. Or maybe, they'll think it's sexy! For supersensitive skins the acidic action of the tomato or papaya may be an irritant.

Yeast and Wheat Germ Oil Mask

Combine 1 tablespoon of powdered brewer's yeast with ½ teaspoon of wheat germ oil. This should make a paste. If it's not the consistency you like, add more oil. Leave it on your face for 10 to 15 minutes, then wash it off with warm water. Apply some of the oil to your face before going to bed. If your face is very dry, use it twice a week.

I hope you'll try one of these baths when you feel the need to rejuvenate your skin all over:

Baking Soda Bath

A half cup of baking soda added to your bathwater will soothe irritated skin and will be a delight on a hot summer day.

Bath Oils

Dry, itchy skin will be relieved by adding baby oil, olive oil, or commercial bath oil to your bath. It takes only a few drops, but you should soak for at least ten minutes to ensure optimum moisturizing. Be careful when climbing in and out of the tub—this makes surfaces very slippery!

Cucumber Bath

Boil unpeeled cucumber slices in a little water to make a juice. Strain the liquid from the pulp. Combine the juice with an equal amount of *glycerin,* and pour 2 tablespoons of the liquid into your bathwater.

Honey Bath

Lia Schorr, the renowned skin-care expert, suggests adding a tablespoon of honey to your bath. It will leave your skin feeling soft and smooth.

HANDS AND FEET

Your hands and feet have special needs. They do a disproportionate share of the skin's work; your hands seem always to be busy and so do your feet, poor soles. All four (two hands, two feet) of them deserve tender care. Hands have less fatty tissue than any other part of the body, and the palms have no oil glands, according to Lia Schorr. So protect them by wearing gloves when housecleaning, gardening, and dishwashing. Keep them well moisturized. Both hands and feet benefit from a petroleum jelly treatment. Lavishly apply it and slip on gloves and socks before going to bed at night. The extremities will be appreciably softer and smoother in the morning. If your feet are callused, soak them in hot water for about 15 minutes, and use a pumice stone on the hardened areas, such as the heels and the balls of the feet. Moisturize them with a rich cream afterward, because the pumice stone, although a gentle abrasive, is still an abrasive.

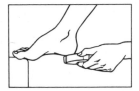

Hand Softeners

A hand softener need not be complicated. Certain basic ingredients can be pulled out of the cupboard or the refrigerator and used almost as is to make hands soft and supple. Olive oil is a good emollient, as is cocoa butter, or a combination of equal parts lanolin and petroleum jelly liberally rubbed into the hands after they have been immersed in water. Soaking hands in a bowl of fresh milk, buttermilk, or water mixed with oatmeal or bran also helps to soothe and smooth them when they are rough and red.

Rose Water and Glycerin Lotion
Mix ½ teaspoon of borax into 1 cup of rose water until it dissolves. Add this mixture to 1 cup of glycerin, stirring constantly. This lotion will smooth and soften hands.

SO WHAT'S A WRINKLE?

Well, my first were crow's feet or laugh lines, whichever name you prefer. (I prefer laugh lines.) If you were to examine your skin under a microscope, you would see that it is covered with an intricate pattern of fine lines. As the skin ages and becomes drier, these lines tend to become deeper. As the skin's support system of collagen and elastin lessens, wrinkles appear. These can become sags and crevices in your face. Note that lines are expressive signs of character, says Lia Schorr. "We will get wrinkles as we get older." What you don't want are crevices caused by deep collagen fiber destruction, from misuse of the sun (note how I put it).

At the same time, the number of new cells being produced in the epidermis tapers off; new cell production may be 30 to 50 percent slower than when you were young. The new cells are larger, thinner, and harder to detach from the surface, according to Dr. Kligman. So, the natural process of sloughing off dead cells, so vital to revealing the fresh, glowing skin beneath, becomes slower and more erratic.

What can be done about the onslaught of wrinkles aside from limiting sun exposure, using appropriate sunscreens, and moisturizing frequently? Wrinkle-fighting is a full-time profession for many skin doctors. Dr. Marvin Brodey, a New York City dermatologist, says, "I could make a lot of money if I wanted to delve into the cosmetic business." One relatively new technique is the injection of natural collagen into the skin. Injected collagen (extracted from cowhide and purified) replaces collagen lost as skin ages, plumping up creases and wrinkles temporarily. However, this injected collagen eventually dissolves, calling for touch-ups every few months. Doctors have mixed feelings about this remedy for wrinkles—some are pleased with the effects; others feel injections are expensive and a waste of time. If I were considering collagen injections, I'd be sure to consult a dermatologist or plastic surgeon who had a lot of experience with the technique.

Another method that is used to repair aging due to the sun is the use of Retin A (retinoic acid, a derivative of vitamin A). "Retin A is not a face-lift, not a face peel," says Dr. Kligman, who has conducted a major study on retinoic acid at the University of Pennsylvania. "It won't remove big-time sagging under the eyes or chin," he adds. "But it will build up the collagen and give the skin a better quality. It can improve the skin's texture, make it fuller, increase its blood vessels, improve its color, and remove small lines and small wrinkles," says Dr. Kligman.

The kind of skin Retin A can help is the one that has been photo-aged (meaning it has been exposed to too much sun). This overexposure to ultraviolet rays causes the skin to become mottled, scaly, and dry. It can also cause pigmentation problems and small wrinkles around the mouth and in the cheeks. Retin A goes to work on these problems. "But the sagging under the eyes and chin that comes from the natural effects of gravity, your constitution, and heredity—the lines that come from laughing or perpetual frowning—can't be changed by Retin A," Dr. Kligman told me. "The drapery of the skin can only be corrected by surgery, and deep wrinkles can only be removed by dermabrasion."

It's entirely possible that Retin A will be sold over the counter within the next five years. But, even now, many dermatologists are prescribing it for its original use, which is to help relieve acne. "You wash your face and apply it," says Dr. Kligman. The only recognizable side effect at this point is that it tends to make the skin more sun sensitive.

COSMETIC SURGERY AND DERMABRASION

Many women at 40 plus consider cosmetic surgery as an option. But even though it is cosmetic, it is *still* surgery. And surgery, no matter what kind, is not to be taken lightly. Lifting a face, breasts, or eyelids is a matter of removing the loose tissue by actually making an incision in the skin and taking out the fat by one of a number of methods. The results of these operations last an average of seven to ten years, sometimes even longer. Bear in mind that although a face-lift will remove the double chin or the heavy jowl, if your skin has a tendency to wrinkle, it will continue to do so.

Doctors use dermabrasion as another way to confront localized skin problems. Deep scars from acne or injury, skin discoloration, furrows in the upper lip area, and crow's feet around the eyes are all frequently treated with dermabrasion, which is just what it sounds like: abrasion that removes skin. Dermabrasion and, similarly, the chemical peel (which burns off the skin's outer layers) are uncomfortable treatments and are recommended only for people who have consulted with their doctors about alternative possibilities and still see one of these measures as the best choice.

SUN AND SKIN

I have had wonderful days on beaches from the south of France to the Virgin Islands, from Malibu to Bridgehampton, from Muscle Beach to Jones Beach, from a beach on Cape Cod to a small stretch of beach on a little island in Maine. I'm sure you have your beach memories, too.

If we could turn back the clock, would any of us have skipped those days on the sand in order to have perfect skin now? I doubt it. Everyone told us that we needed the "rays" anyway (vitamin D, and all that). No one said that the sun was a direct assault on our collagen and elastin, the duo that keeps our skin firm.

Facts about Face-lifts and Other Cosmetic Surgery

Cosmetic Procedure	Complications	Comments
Eyelids and Bags (Blepharoplasty) Eliminates droopy eyelids, bags under eyes caused by heredity, age, sleeplessness, alcohol, stress; can be performed as an outpatient	Blood clots, temporary blindness, turned-out lower lid	Popular procedure because it offers youthful look; scar concealed in upper-lid crease; lasts 10 to 15 years
Face-lift (Rhytidectomy) Removal of excessive skin from face and neck; hospital stay usually required; continuous sunscreen protection prescribed; may require additional procedures*	Hematoma (blood under skin), paralyzed nerves, infection	Removes 10 to 20 years, but not fine lines; dark circles are not affected; lasts 5 to 10 years; facial habits may cause frown line and wrinkles to reappear; patients should be prepared for a postoperative letdown
Nose Reshaping (Rhinoplasty) Building, reducing or reconstructing nose; performed in a hospital with two-week recovery	Swelling and black eyes; may take weeks for nose to take on final shape	Scars are inside nose; may activate latent allergies; not recommended for people with distorted self-images

*Removal of crow's feet, lines in upper lip, or acne scars requires dermabrasion (sandblasts the skin) or chemical peel (burns off the skin layers); both are painful and may leave skin mottled. Collagen is a natural substance injected into skin as a cheaper nonsurgical alternative, but it is absorbed by the body and lasts only a few months or so.

Now that I'm 49, I *am* taking certain precautions. I stay out of the noonday sun. I wear a sunscreen, put zinc oxide (that thick white stuff) on my nose, and never use a reflector.

It can't be denied; the sun is the *number one* cause of premature aging of the skin. This means that it contributes to wrinkles, loss of tone, sagging, and a tough, dry texture. To make matters worse, sun exposure has been scientifically proven to promote skin cancer.

It was recently reported by the American Cancer Society that one out of every seven Americans has skin cancer. Generally, it is brought on from overexposure to the sun over a period of many years. The superficial skin cancers can be detected by a physician easily and early on, and cancers of this type almost always respond to treatment. Melanoma is a grave form of skin cancer, and doctors recommend checking on any change in size, color, shape, thickness, or texture of moles, beauty marks, or dark pigment patches.

WHAT HAPPENS WHEN SUN MEETS SKIN

Sun is an agent provocateur where skin is involved. The familiar lobster-red burn, often the skin's first reaction to the sun, comes from the immediate trauma of massive dilation of your skin's blood vessels. A suntan is the skin's way of protecting itself, of shielding itself from further damage. Each square inch of the epidermis, or the outer layer of the skin, contains thousands of the cells (melanocytes) that produce malanin pigment when exposed to ultraviolet radiation. And that's how you get a suntan.

Also, the older you are, the more vulnerable your skin is to showing those little, unsightly dark patches, often known as liver spots, or age spots. These have nothing to do with liver; they are brought on by the sun. Other by-products of sun exposure are very taut, dehydrated skin; rashes; and itchy, uncomfortable skin.

Most middle-aged women are particularly fearful of solar elastosis, the technical name given to the loss of skin elasticity due to the sun. Continued exposure to ultraviolet rays damages the elastic fibers in the dermis, the part of the skin beneath the surface. Once elasticity is lost, wrinkles can become indelibly etched into the skin. This condition builds up over the years, so its ravaging effects become more obvious with age. Damage that has been done cannot be reversed, but increased damage can be avoided, and the signs of aging can be retarded by using a little common sense. Bear in mind, while I say this, that sun damage does not harm everyone the same way at the same time. Much depends on the individual skin type and on how quickly you tan or burn. The darker your skin is to begin with, the better off you will be in the face of chronic sun exposure. Blacks and olive-skinned people have the relative advantage of skin already darkened with the protective melanin pigment, which will absorb some of the harmful ultraviolet rays.

A WORD ABOUT SUNLAMPS AND TANNING SALONS

Convenience, trendiness, and a relatively inexpensive price tag all help to account for the popularity of artificial tanning. It is the refuge of some women, but such measures are to be avoided like poison. The use of artificial light may be a staggering ten times the ultraviolet radiation than that from a midday summer sun. Many quick-tan aficionados have suffered from severe burns and painful eye irritations.

HOW TO HANDLE THE SUN

Now that I've scared you about exposure to the sun, let me tell you this: I love the sun. This may be anathema to say in skin-care circles, but truthfully, I wouldn't give it up completely even if I could have beautiful skin like the actress Molly Ringwald's. I grew up on the beaches of California (where sun-worshiping is an everyday ritual), and my husband and I would not give up our yearly Caribbean vacation in St. John for anything in the world. But I have learned that to enjoy the sun and still care for my skin properly, I must exercise a good deal of caution. And these days I do.

I don't stay in the sun as long as I used to. I certainly avoid exposure to it between 12:00 and 2:00 P.M. When I'm feeling too parched, I get under a shade tree (in St. John) or an umbrella (at Jones Beach). I've invested in a wide-brimmed straw hat and sunglasses. I use SPF #15 sunscreen. And as I've said, I put zinc oxide on my nose or it would turn the color of a radish, with more broken capillaries than I would care to think about. I *don't* sunburn anymore. I don't even get as much of a tan as I used to get. But I still get out in the sun.

I know there are those who say I should stay off the beach completely and maybe even carry a parasol on any summer day. But I bolster myself with the words of Dr. Brodey, who says: "The ultraviolet rays of the sun do damage . . . but I won't tell people to stay out of the sun if they love the sun. You might as well enjoy yourself and live while you're alive because you'll be under the ground a long time. But you don't have to roast, and you should never use a reflector. You should stay out of the sun at high noon and use sunscreens. Use common sense, but for heaven's sake, live!"

And live I do, but with a little more caution, at least about the noonday sun.

WHAT NOT TO DO IN THE SUN

I certainly don't recommend avoiding the sun entirely, in pursuit of a china-doll pallor. That's not my style; I prefer a healthy glow. I love being outdoors, exercising and enjoying the elements. But you don't have to be an accomplice to the sun's damaging rays. Take these simple measures:

✔ **Avoid the sun at its hottest, strongest, and when it's deceptive.**

Be aware of the sun's differing strengths at different times of the day. The sun is most intense between 11:00 A.M. and 3:00 P.M. (I cheat by an hour and get back under it by 2:00 P.M., but I wear my sun hat.) In midsummer, you can enjoy the hot sun before and after those hours and still pick up color. Look out for seaside and poolside factors that actually conspire to increase the sun's burning potential. Sand and concrete (and for the skiers—snow) can all exacerbate the sun's damage by reflecting sunlight. And a cloudy day is no license to bask on the beach unprotected. Just because you can't see the sun does not mean it isn't there. It's still up there, blazing away, and the clouds do little to absorb the ultraviolet rays that can burn your skin.

✔ **Avoid perfumes, cosmetics, deodorants, and certain drugs while exposed to the sun.**

This doesn't apply to everyone, but it is a good, general rule of thumb. Many people are sensitive to the interaction between ultraviolet rays and a wide range of commonly used chemicals and ingredients either consumed or applied to the skin. The result is an annoying itch or rash. Among the more widespread troublemakers are certain oils used in perfumes: oil of bergamot, lemon, lime, lavender, sandalwood, and cedar. Other offenders are saccharin (in low-calorie foods and beverages), hexachlorophene (used in many deodorant and cosmetic preparations), and certain medica-tions, including tetracycline and diuretics. Surprisingly, some natural foods can be photo-sensitizing substances; the list includes celery, figs, parsnips, citrus fruits, and vanilla. So, if you find yourself itching uncomfortably on the beach, that vanilla ice cream, lemonade, or diet cola you just gulped down might have something to do with it.

✔ **Don't depend on the water to protect you.**

The rays of the sun burn right through the water. You can get a sunburn while swimming underwater because "the weakening of ultraviolet light by water is almost zero," according to Dr. Kligman. It is best to wear a waterproof sunscreen. In fact sunscreens are a major weapon in slowing the aging process of your skin, according to Dr. Kligman. Unless you're a fisherman who's constantly exposed, you can go out in the sun and have little damage if you use SPF #15.

✔ **Never, never use a sun reflector.**

That is, unless you want to dramatically speed up the aging process.

WHAT TO DO IN THE SUN

Here are some basics to help keep you comfortable and safe in the sun:

✔ **Keep yourself hydrated.**

Drink lots and lots of fluids, especially water. This is important all year-round, rain or shine. Drinking six to eight glasses of water a day will keep your skin hydrated, help your digestion, and slake your thirst. Spray water on yourself several times over the course of a day in the sun; I like those spray bottles and carry one with me to the beach.

✔ **Seek shade when the sun begins to feel oppressive.**

Umbrellas, shady trees, and awnings are there to be used like I use my favorite tree at Majo Bay beach. One caveat, however: Shade does not mean total protection. It often reduces sun exposure by no more than half, so seek out the shade, but for complete protection, invest in a wide-brimmed hat, a cotton cover-up (a good-looking caftan), and good-quality sunglasses. "A woman of 80 could look like most kids at 25 if she takes care of her skin and doesn't go in the sun, or covers her skin with sunscreen," says Dr. Kligman. "The skin on your bottom is not usually exposed to the sun and you can see the good shape it is in."

✔ **Slather on sunscreens.**

I strongly urge you not to be stingy in using sunscreens. They come in a choice of oils, creams, gels, and lotions, with a number that signifies their strength. The best screens contain PABA (para-aminobenzoic acid), zinc oxide, or titanium oxide.

PABA and related chemicals work by creating a chemical shield against the ultraviolet rays. Opaque sunblocks like zinc oxide and titanium oxide provide a physical barrier between your skin and the sun. Both sunscreens and sunblocks have critically enhanced the lives of many sun lovers, like me, because they are tremendously effective when used properly. They should be applied at least *30 minutes* before going out in the sun and generously *reapplied* all day, particularly after swimming or perspiring. If you have very sensitive skin, many doctors recommend testing a sunscreen on a small patch of skin a day or two before you plan to use it to make sure it doesn't cause a rash.

SUNSCREENS: HOW TO KNOW WHAT TO USE

The U.S. Food and Drug Administration has established a standard sun protection system based on skin types. The six categories are:

1. Sun sensitive—Skin always burns, never tans.

2. Sun sensitive—Skin burns easily, tans minimally.

3. Normal—Skin burns moderately, tans gradually.

4. Normal—Skin burns minimally, always tans well.

5. Insensitive—Skin rarely burns, tans deeply.

6. Insensitive—Skin never burns, tans profusely.

After identifying your correct skin type, you should pick the sunscreen that will work best for you:

✔ SPF 15 or greater—ultra protection

✔ SPF 8 to 15—strong protection

✔ SPF 4 to 8—moderate protection

✔ SPF 2 to 4—minimum protection

The numbers in the grading system indicate how long you can stay out in the sun with that specific protection factor. For example, an SPF of 8 means you can spend eight hours in the sun and theoretically absorb only one hour's worth of rays.

But the sunscreen can wash off with perspiration or swimming, so look for one that's waterproof. And reapply it often. Dermatologists say that even so-called waterproof products don't always adhere as well in real life as they do in the lab.

Coping with the sun is simply a matter of common sense. Use your own good judgment to protect your skin.

What Can Be Done about Age Spots and the Like?

Age spots, the brown patches caused by sun exposure, are hard to deal with. I'm sure you have heard about miracle fade creams and bleaches, but before you invest your money in such remedies, there are a few things to know about them.

For starters, they do (yes!) work. But not the way we would like them to. They work very, very slowly, and the results are often only temporary. The most effective creams of this type will contain the active ingredient hydroquinine. It is safe to use, but it doesn't really bleach the spot; instead it inhibits the production of melanin, or pigment. So the lower-level cells, which are making the trek to the outer layer, won't be carrying their normal load of pigment. This process can take a long time, and you have to use the creams *twice a day, regularly.* If you stop using the creams, the spots often come back.

New developments have been made recently in the field of laser surgery. This technique can be used to permanently fade the age spots and to remove spider veins, but it should be carefully considered. Not only is it costly but there can be complications, like scarring, loss of pigmentation, or even a permanent depression in the skin where the spot was.

AND WHAT'S MORE: THE TRIED AND TRUE BASICS

A look in the mirror tells me I'll never be 20, 30, or even 40 again. But, as you may have guessed by now, I'm happy to be where I am. It has taken me years and hard work to build the character I have today, and I think my face shows it. That's the best cosmetic I could ask for. Lia Schorr gave me a boost in that direction when she said, "Wrinkles? They're not wrinkles, they're character lines, the demarcations that lend depth and wisdom to the face." But I do want to have the best possible skin at my age, I won't kid you about that. So I follow these tried and true health basics, just as conscientiously as I now slather on my Lubriderm and my sunscreens.

BASIC NUMBER ONE: DRINK PLENTY OF WATER

I can't overstress the importance of water. Lots of water contributes to your total well-being. Drinking six to eight glasses daily is essential to maintaining bodily moisture. Put lemon in it (vitamin C, too!) if you have trouble drinking that much water straight.

BASIC NUMBER TWO: GET ENOUGH SLEEP

Nothing shows itself in your appearance so quickly as a lack of sleep. A poor night's sleep is written all over the face, leaving its evidence with puffy eyes, a sallow complexion, and a lackluster look. Sleep seven to eight hours a night in a cool, dark room with fresh air when possible. (Remember the green plants!) Establish good habits of going to bed at roughly the same time each night, and avoid stimulants and alcohol before bedtime.

BASIC NUMBER THREE: EAT A HEALTHFUL DIET

Without good nutrition your body loses its ability to ward off illness and infections. Such a systemic breakdown has effects on your whole body, not just your face. Maintaining your health depends on meeting your body's requirement for vitamins (get enough A, B, C, and E, especially for your skin), minerals, and nutrients. "After 40, it's especially important to watch liquor, wine, and coffee intake, drug use, smoking, and spicy and sweet foods," says Lia Schorr. "Avoid sugar, eat whole wheat breads, chicken, fish, and vegetables." Eat well (read the diet section once more) and your skin will thank you for it!

BASIC NUMBER FOUR: EXERCISE REGULARLY AND OFTEN

"Exercise is good for skin," says Dr. Kligman. "It increases the blood supply to the skin, so you'll look rosier. Measurements of athletes' skin show that it tends to be thicker; the collagen tends to remain thicker," he adds. Exercise promotes good circulation, which ensures that your blood will be carrying oxygen to all the hard-to-reach places. Adequate exercise will keep your skin glowing and may even give you some surprising bonuses. Several doctors have reported that bags under the eyes will gradually disappear with regular exercise, and that the skin's ability to replenish itself will be greatly improved.

BASIC NUMBER FIVE: ELIMINATE SMOKING

We all know smoking is no life extender. We're all familiar with the dangers to our heart and lungs from smoking. But to our skin? When a smoker inhales, the lips crease into vertical lines and the eyes narrow. These wrinkle-prone areas simply don't need any more aggravation, which smoking causes. Additionally, nicotine causes the skin's small blood vessels to contract, and that inhibits circulation. This shows itself in the dull pallor and excessive wrinkles often seen in the faces of many smokers at mid-life.

BASIC NUMBER SIX: LIMIT ALCOHOL INTAKE

Drinking too much brings on dark pouches under the eyes, reddish spider veins on the cheeks and around the nose, and a general dehydrated skin condition. It's a good idea, after a drink or two, to replenish the moisture you've lost to alcohol with lots of water.

BASIC NUMBER SEVEN: AVOID CRASH DIETS

Crash dieters often suffer from flabby skin, wrinkles, and drooping breasts. Worst of all is on-and-off dieting; the repeated gaining and losing damages your skin in a peculiar way. When skin is stretched and shrunk time and again, it tends to lose its elasticity. Remember, on the Turn-Back-the-Clock Diet, you're supposed to lose only two pounds a week.

BASIC NUMBER EIGHT: AVOID FACIAL EXERCISES AND EXAGGERATED EXPRESSIONS

Both exercises and expressions overwork your skin. Have you ever noticed how some people appear to have a scowl permanently etched into their faces? This comes from scrunching up the skin too often. Try to keep your face and skin relaxed. Well, try most of the time. Publishers' deadlines tend to make me frown, and I'm sure you have your Achilles' heel as well.

So before we move on to the next chapter, let me clue you in on this book's credo, if you haven't caught on yet. You may not be able to prevent the years from rollin' in and addin' up, but you *can* look like the best version of *yourself* right now, right where you are in *your* life.

WHEN GRAY HAIR IS GREAT & WHEN IT'S NOT

Chapter 4

When I think about hair, I think of my grandmother and my Aunt Dorothy. My grandmother said if you had good hair and good shoes, everything else fell into place. In Aunt Dorothy's philosophy of life, hair came first. "You're only as good as your hair," she said. Aunt Dorothy bleached her hair blonde and wore it over one eye like Veronica Lake, who was known to movie-goers of the forties as the Peek-a-Boo Girl. Because those were the days when only movie stars were brazen enough to dye their hair and admit it, we could only guess about Aunt Dorothy's wicked habit, but I'd say it was a sure-shot guess. Coloring was not so great in those days.

When I think of hair, I also think of the movie *Educating Rita,* in which a young English female hairdresser "betters" herself by studying literature with a kind, but alcoholic professor. In a scene set in Rita's beauty parlor, a heavy, plain, way-past-40 woman holds up a movie magazine picture of Princess Di. "That's what I want to look like," she tells Rita.

The women in the audience laughed—haven't we all done something like that at one time or another? How easy to see someone else look foolish when she's trying to look like someone she bears not the slightest resemblance to. Well, Princess Di wasn't around when we were young, but we had our own heroines. (Aunt Dorothy had Veronica Lake; I had Doris Day.) And now? Have we wised up to the realities of the midlife hair crisis? During the midlife hair crisis, many of us still revert to a color and style that isn't us at all—one that is too girlish or too severe or doesn't work with our hair's texture. The result? We look older.

It's easy to make drastic moves at this stage in life (and, in fact, whenever we're uneasy or depressed, we tend to make drastic moves with our hair). But wait. Stop. Think. Look before you leap to scissors, perm, or dye. Your hair may have become gray and even thinner, but frantically curling it to add fullness or covering it up with color may be the wrong thing to do. Teasing plays havoc with ailing hair and so can permanents, if not done properly. And you may want to keep yours gray. Gray is nature's way of creating a soft frame for a complexion that may be losing some of its color. Treated right, gray can be gorgeous (as you'll see in one of the makeovers in this chapter).

HEALTHY, SHINY HAIR IS THE GOAL

Hair grows out of follicles in the scalp. Eighty-five percent of your hair is growing most of the time. The rest is either between growing stages or about to fall out. Every one of those hairs has a life cycle of three to ten years. On an average hair grows at a rate of one-half inch per month, making it about two years old when it is a foot long. During that time your hair can take a lot of abuse—and that wear and tear can affect how it looks and behaves.

We have to combat the enemies of healthy hair: harsh weather conditions, crash dieting (especially too severe a cutback in protein and iron that usually accompanies very low-calorie diets), stress, vitamin megadoses, certain drugs, hormonal changes brought on by menopause, perming, straightening, teasing, and too vigorous brushing (holdover from the "100 strokes a day" advice from our grandmothers and relatives like Aunt Dorothy).

What can you do for this poor, weather-beaten, twisted, and tugged hair? Here's what.

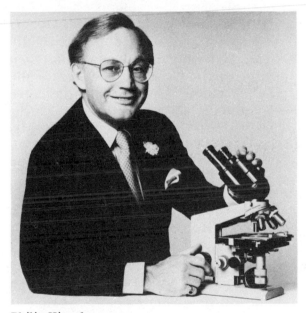

Philip Kingsley

Philip Kingsley, a trained trichologist (a specialist in scalp and hair science) and author of *The Complete Hair Book* (New York: Grosset & Dunlap, 1979), believes that "healthy hair is a combination of a healthy body and sensible hair care." We talked with him at the Philip Kingsley Trichological Center in New York City:

"The best way to make sure your hair is in good condition is to eat properly and exercise regularly," he said. "Excessive animal fat, excessive salt, and excessive sugar are terrible for your health and terrible for your hair." On the other hand, he feels that plenty of fruits, fresh vegetables, whole grains, salads, plus lean fish and poultry are great for your hair and health. You should also drink eight glasses of water a day. (Remember this is good for your skin as well.)

"Exercise helps circulation and is relaxing," said Mr. Kingsley. If you get the feeling that exercise is good for everything, you're right. And if you think that what's good for one part of the body is good for almost all the others, you're right again. To repeat what Mr. Kingsley says, "healthy hair requires a healthy body."

You aren't healthy if you are under inappropriate stress (but, as Dr. Hans Selye, who was the foremost expert on stress once said, you have to decide what is appropriate for you). One of the places the effects of too much stress show up is in the condition of your hair. "Dandruff acts up when women are under special stress," said Mr. Kingsley. "Sometimes stress causes hair loss, although it can also be caused by underlying problems like anemia, thyroid, or gynecological problems."

Stress probably speeds graying. In support of this theory, researchers have reported experiments in which the hair of black rats turned white when they were put on diets deficient in B (the "nerve") vitamins. When they were again given B vitamins, their hair turned black. Since the body uses up more vitamin B when it's under stress, it is reasonable to conclude that stress could have an effect on the graying of hair. So, Mr. Kingsley recommends his clients take B vitamins and also suggests they take brewer's yeast every day—for dry hair take vitamin E and cod-liver oil tablets. For a woman who might be suffering from anemia, he suggests iron in the form of defatted liver tablets, plus a good iron supplement.

Does menopause affect the hair? Does your hair continue to grow after menopause? Mr. Kingsley told me that if a woman has a family history of thinning hair during menopause, her own hair may thin a little bit. But by the average age of menopause, say 50, a woman would not have hair as thick as when she was 27 anyway. In fact, no woman over 40 has the volume of hair she did when she was in her twenties and thirties.

As the skin ages, the hair follicles age, becoming slightly smaller in diameter. So although the woman would have a similar number of hairs, they would probably be thinner in diameter, giving the appearance and feeling of less hair. As for balding, Mr. Kingsley said it is unlikely that a woman will bald as a man balds, although the amount of thinning in women is almost as high as in men. But you don't get complete baldness. Women suffer from volume loss. Whether or not thinning is slight or considerable really depends upon genetic predisposition just as it does with men. And balding, if you'll remember, is inherited from your mother's genes.

Most damaged follicles are the result of excessive hair brushing. Hair dyes do cause some damage, said Mr. Kingsley, but less so these

Candice Robins on Perms, Mousses, Medications, and Hot Rollers

The Last Word on Perms

"If a permanent wave is done well, it can be a great asset to your appearance," says Candice. "People should look at perms more creatively than they do, planning them to harmonize with the shape of the face for best effect. A perm shouldn't be used to correct hair problems but to create curl." Generally, if the hair is healthy, the perm will be good; but a perm can play havoc with damaged hair. That's simply because damaged hair doesn't tolerate chemicals well. Here are factors you should think about before you get a perm.

✔ If it's body or volume you want, you can get it through a good haircut. Don't use a perm to compensate for a bad haircut or to disguise unhealthy hair. Think of a perm as an ornament like lipstick.

✔ Perms are hard on the hair due to all those chemicals. Don't have a perm more than twice a year.

✔ If the hair is at all damaged, you get a lot of breakage from a perm. I don't recommend perms for hair that has been colored.

✔ A perm should be rolled loosely. Most problems with perms are the result of too-tight wrapping. If rolled too tightly in a square pattern (across the top, straight down the back, and straight down the sides), it pulls because hair doesn't grow that way. Natural hair patterns are not rigidly geometric. Remember, the idea of a perm is to mimic a natural curl.

✔ A perm is a chemical process, so the operator must watch the timing carefully. You should have an experienced person to do your perm.

✔ Partial perms are great. You might just perm the top of the head, or just the sides, or just the back. Since people have different textures of hair at different places on their heads (sometimes curly in one place and not the other), perms can be planned to equalize the curl in the hair.

A Matter of Mousse

Candice says that "mousses are used in the same way gels are used. As you know, dirty hair is easier to handle than clean hair; clean hair is slippery. A mousse makes hair gooey; that's why people like to work with it. Hair with mousse on it tends to stay put. Use mousse on dry hair to place it, then let the mousse dry and it will hold unless you disturb it with your hands.

(continued)

Candice Robins on Perms, Mousses, Medications, and Hot Rollers—*Continued*

"I don't like mousses," she says. "I think they are a big gimmick, although I know mousses are appealing, even fun, to apply—like Crazy Foam in the bathtub.

"One reason many beauty experts do use mousses: By eliminating the need to blow-dry certain hairstyles into place, you are less likely to dry out your hair—a common problem with older hair."

What about Medications?

How do medications affect the hair? Anything that affects circulation or the general health of the body affects the hair. So prolonged use of aspirin, birth control pills, cortisone, and other medications can cause an itchy, inflamed scalp or hair loss. Once you stop the medication, the scalp itch or hair loss usually stops.

The Case for Hot Rollers

Do hot rollers, those electrically heated curlers that wave your hair in minutes, damage the hair? "Not necessarily," says Candice. "The older types with metal or plastic spiked rods did cause pulls and tangles, but the newer models avoid that. Today hot rollers are made with a soft surface that cradles your hair, protecting the hair from coming into contact with the hot inner core of the rod."

days, as the formulas are better now. Some actually condition and enhance your hair. As for the cancer scare a few years ago concerning hair dyes, later studies showed that the concerns were seriously exaggerated. "I think the hair dyes now are rather good," he said. One note of caution, "progressive" dyes still contain lead acetate, a toxin absorbed by the skin.

The more things you do to your hair, the more you need to compensate by conditioning and massaging. Fortunately the new products are less damaging and that includes electric hair rollers on the market in the last two or three years. "Electric hair rollers are an unfortunate necessity," said Mr. Kingsley. "The new ones aren't so bad. They are thermostated and they let out a little steam, which doesn't dry the hair up as much as the old ones. If a woman wants to use hot rollers, she should, bearing in mind that she is adding problems onto problems if her hair is already overprocessed by chemicals or heat products.

Brushing can damage hair. Brushing is said to stimulate the scalp and to an extent that's true—but proper massage stimulates the scalp much better, said Mr. Kingsley. What heavy brushing does do is break the hair and pull it out and scratch the scalp, he added. "I'm not saying don't brush at all. But don't use brushing in place of a good sawtooth comb. Rather brush to smooth the hair as a final step in hair grooming. And don't let the bristles dig into the scalp."

To counteract any further shrinking of hair follicles that cause volume loss or thinning (and deal with overprocessed hair at the same time), you need to take care of your scalp. It's not too late even if you're past 50. What you do, advised Mr. Kingsley, is the following:

- ✔ Wash your hair every day.

- ✔ Condition your hair. Once or twice a week, apply a deep remoisturizing conditioner 30 minutes before washing. Then condition your hair. On other days, simply condition after shampooing.

- ✔ Don't brush your hair. Gently comb it with a sawtooth comb.

- ✔ Eat a diet that includes foods rich in B vitamins, such as whole grain cereals, dairy foods, nuts and seeds, organ meats, and fish.

- ✔ Exercise.

- ✔ Eat a healthful diet.

FOUR MAGICAL MAKEOVERS FROM THREE SPINNERS OF MAGIC

I have known two women who improved their looks enormously by letting "their hair go gray." One had dyed her hair red for years. It was overprocessed and never matched her complexion or her personality. Once she let the gray come out, her skin had a heightened color and she, in fact, looked years younger. Her gray hair, which she wore short, was thick and had a wonderfully silvery "salt and pepper" look.

The other woman had dyed her hair black. It was one of those shoe-polish blacks, which made her skin look pale and pasty. Once she let her lovely, thick, silver hair grow out, her skin came alive as the other woman's had. Her hair was silvery, the color Barbara Stanwyck has now. She wore it a medium length, looked chic and glamorous, whereas before she had looked hard.

Keeping your gray hair is usually the best choice. But hair colorist Walter Chadwick says, "It's time to give up on gray when the color doesn't complement the tones of the skin, and the placement of gray is uneven and unflattering." Then you should go for highlights or an all-over color change with a good colorist; doing your own is a disaster.

In the four magical makeovers that follow, you'll see how—and why—each hairstyle and/or change in color flatters and lifts years from the face. Cheaper and quicker than a face-lift, these "befores and afters" will clearly show how remarkably rejuvenating the right hairstyle can be.

Stylist Candice Robins of David Daines Hair Salon on Madison Avenue is a chatty, witty woman of 32, who is also a sculptor with a degree in fine arts. She started styling hair to "make a living" and has now fallen in love with the art. She approaches each individual's head of hair as though she were a sculptor. "It is very exciting for me to see the changes that are made in women's lives by changing their hair," said Candice. "They'll call me back and say, 'I can't keep the men away now,' or 'I'm moving to California.' There is nothing worse than bad hair," said Candice. "You take off your makeup and your clothes, but when you're naked, you've still got your hair."

Walter Chadwick, also of David Daines Hair Salon, is a soft-spoken, thoughtful man in his early twenties, whose art training was in photography. He also has an artist's approach to hair color. He loves color, but color that is natural looking. "The mistake made by many women who color their own hair is that they come up with unnatural-looking hair colors—colors that give hair coloring a bad name. There should be no standard hair colors but mixtures that emulate nature. There is no right or wrong hair color: Gray is not all bad, nor is all brown hair drab. It depends on how the head of hair looks altogether—its depth, its highlights. Hair you dye yourself tends to be flat—all one color, unlike the variegated hair color women get from nature. I don't believe in assembly-line color. And that, unfortunately, is just what I see too much of.

Gigi Williams, 36, is a makeup stylist for TV and magazine personalities. She spins her magic from one small makeup kit. A rapid-fire talker with a keen wit, Gigi doesn't think women need to fuss a lot with their makeup. They should take a makeup lesson and learn to correctly apply their makeup. Then they'll become so skilled they can put it on in a few minutes. Gigi said she can tell how old a woman is by her makeup and hairstyle. "Usually most of us are learning to fix our hair and apply makeup when we are between 18 and 21, at the height of our narcissism," she said. "That's the time we often get stuck with our makeup for life. My own mother still wears her lipstick, eyeliner, and hairstyle just as she did in the 1950s. But what seemed to look good at one stage of life may have long since ceased to be right for you."

These three "magicians" did the four magical makeovers in this chapter. If you ever doubted that all of us can be the best, most beautiful versions of ourselves, doubt no more. Read through the next few pages and look at the pictures; then make an appointment for yourself at the best hair salon you can find. We'll tell you how later on. Now for our four "swans":

MILENA KRONDL, 43 (photos, page 99)

Milena Before

Milena is single, skis, runs, and plans events for the New York City Road Runner's Club. Eight years ago she came to this country from Czechoslovakia and still has an accent, which adds to her charming European manner. She is tall, adventurous, and very witty. Red is definitely the right color for her hair—but not the red she had. It was in her own words a "frizzy, latter-day hippie look." Candice said that Milena's hair was, well, "brassy." But, as Milena was as candid and outspoken as Candice, who is also a redhead, they got along fine. Anything Candice wanted to do with her hair was fine with Milena. She was "out for adventure." Milena said:

> I have done my own hair color for almost ten years. I dyed it suddenly after losing a job. What kind of hair color do I use? Oh, this or that, whatever I can find. I was born with naturally curly hair but had ironed it for years, until I lost another job (I've only lost two, mind you). Then I got an Afro permanent. Remember those? That Afro jogged my memory. I remembered that my own hair was naturally curly, so I just let my own curl grow out. I keep my hair curly and long because it is easy to care for. I like the freedom of not having to bother with my hair. But I do think my hair is washed out now. It's the color of carrots—and it's so frizzy.

Candice's and Walter's Plan for Milena

"Milena's hair is naturally a medium brown," Candice said. "But red does work well with her skin tone and the blueness of her eyes. It's just the wrong red right now. I would keep her hair red but closer to the shade of her real hair. Long hair suits her personality, but I would trim and shape it.

Milena After
Her Hair

Candice cut off the frizzy, dry ends caused by overprocessing in her home hair-coloring efforts. She also layered Milena's hair to give it more fullness and bounce. Walter mixed a rich auburn shade for Milena which approximated the shade of her original medium brown hair—a tone that naturally complemented her skin tone. "A colorist must aim for this," he explained. He also gave Milena's hair highlights of several shades of red. When you dye your own hair, it tends to come out all one shade (or "dense" in color), not subtly varied like your natural hair, which is not one color but many. Walter's coloration would "imitate" real hair color and cover her hair evenly. He says that home dying often overprocesses hair, drying out the ends, which may appear either too dark or too light.

After Walter finished Milena's color, he allowed her hair to dry naturally. "With curly hair, the less you do the better," said Candice.

Her Makeup

Before Milena got her final comb-out, Gigi applied makeup calculated to complement Milena's new hair color and to bring out Milena's beautiful blue eyes. "She had on horrible blue eye shadow," Gigi said. "If you wear bright-colored eye shadow, it takes away from your eye color. The idea is to focus on your eyes—not on your lids."

Gigi applied a neutral grape shade. She used a little beige base with no tint in it, because Milena's skin is quite ruddy. She shaped Milena's eyebrows by applying a little shaving soap with a small bristle brush, then tweezing out a few hairs underneath. Gigi applied black mascara and black pencil liner on her top eyelid. Because Milena's eyes tended to droop, Gigi stopped the line one-quarter inch from the end of her eyes and drew it upward to her brow bone. Then she smudged it so that you would see only the shading, but no demarcation.

Milena's Reaction

"I love it." Then she looked into the mirror and smiled. "Now my life begins."

GLORIA ZECHE, 48 (photos, page 100) ───────────

Gloria Before

Gloria is an attorney for New York City's Mental Health Information Service. She is single, keeps fit playing tennis and swimming, and loves the theater and opera. Her hair started to turn gray in her early thirties. It was all one length and rather flat on top, and she wore it parted on the side. She wore a little makeup and glasses. At 48, she said she "felt better" than she ever had in her life. But she was reluctant to change her hair color, although she would go for a change in style "as long as it wasn't too radical." Gloria said:

> My hair has been gray for so long I've gotten used to it. And I guess I just accept it, too, because it is different. People remember me because I have gray hair. I also remember that my mother dyed her hair and it looked terrible. I haven't had my hair styled in years, but I do have it trimmed once a month by a guy who comes to my apartment to do it. It's convenient that way.

Candice's and Walter's Plan for Gloria

Both felt that Gloria's particular gray was not attractive—that it was a greenish charcoal shade that drained color from her face. And Candice felt that the one-layer hairstyle dragged down the lines of Gloria's face, making her look much older than she was. After some coaxing, Gloria gave in. "I may never get another chance to see what I look like without the gray," she said.

Gloria After

Her Hair

Walter mixed a rich, red-brown color for Gloria that was a little lighter and certainly brighter than her natural color before "going" gray. He mixed a semipermanent color that would last only six weeks, giving Gloria the opportunity to revert to gray at that point if she so desired. Before Walter applied the color, Candice layered Gloria's hair to give Gloria's own naturally wavy hair a lift. It had been weighted down by its length, and now curls began to pop up here and there. The entire shape and look of Gloria's face seemed to change. Then the color was applied and her hair blown dry and combed. The change, as you can see, was astonishing. Without her weighty gray hair, Gloria seemed to lose ten years of her age.

Her Makeup

Next Gigi went to work. First she arched Gloria's eyebrows, which were too thick, detracted from her eyes, and seemed to pull her face down. Then Gigi used Chanel Bisque (beige) base and a bright rose blusher "to bring color to Gloria's face." Smoky gray and deep purple eye shadow were used on Gloria's eyelids. A black eyeliner pencil was used to outline her upper eyelid. At the outer end of the lid, the eyeliner was drawn upward and smudged at the end. Black mascara was applied. Gloria's lips were outlined with a lip pencil. Then a bright pink lipstick was applied. The makeup looked terrific with her glasses. "Women tend to hide behind their glasses and not wear makeup," said Gigi. "They should pay attention to every detail of their makeup whether they wear glasses or not."

Gloria's Reaction

She borrowed an ear cuff from her friend—a jazzy thing for this lady lawyer to do—and stuck it on her ear for her "after" picture. Then she looked in the mirror and said, "I look so striking." What would the judge say to all this? "Contempt of court," she answered, without batting an eye.

RUTH ANN CRANSTON, 46 (photos, page 101) ————————————

Ruth Ann Before

Ruth Ann, married and the mother of grown children, teaches elementary school. She and her husband recently moved to New York City from Minneapolis. When we met Ruth Ann, she was in the process of growing out an "unbelievably short and horrible" cut she had received four months earlier. Her hair—a medium brown and of a fine texture—was one length and emphasized her broad jawline. It was also too flat on top. The overall effect was to make Ruth Ann look wilted. "People who have fine hair always think a blunt cut is best, but they're wrong," said Candice. "Hair like that needs layering to give the impression of volume." Ruth Ann says:

> As a kid in high school, I wore a ponytail and bangs. In college, my hair was sort of long and straight. Since then, I've found out my hair does look better short because it's so straight. The last three years are the longest I've ever gone without a perm since my college years, and I can manage without one. After I turned 40, I didn't notice any particular change in my hair. There's no gray to speak of, but if and when my hair turns gray, I'm going to color it because I don't think it will be a pretty gray. I'm still smarting from the cut and color I got last March. I went to a salon a friend told me about. The stylist butchered my hair and gave me a henna rinse that turned my hair flaming red. I left the shop in tears. I ran home and called another beauty salon to see if they could fix it. They said yes, they could take me that afternoon. There was nothing they could do about taking the color out, but blonde highlights would soften the brassiness. I came out looking fairly presentable. Why am I here after all that? I'm still hoping for a style that flatters me—one I can manage myself without frequent trips to the hairdresser.

(continued on page 103)

NEW HAIRDO, NEW YOU!

Milena Krondl, 43

Long hair suited Milena, but the frizzy dry ends were cut and the hair was layered to provide more fullness and bounce. Red was the right color for Milena's hair, but she had the wrong shade for her skin tone and eyes. She was given a rich auburn shade that was closer to her own natural medium brown, plus highlights of several shades of red. A new makeup complemented the new hair color and her beautiful blue eyes—a beige base with no tint, natural grape eye shadow with black mascara, and black pencil liner on the top lid. "I love it," said Milena. "Now my life begins."

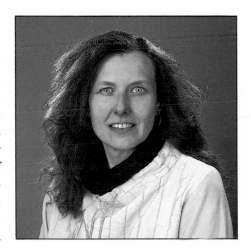

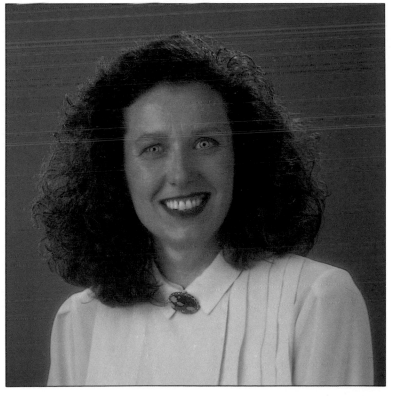

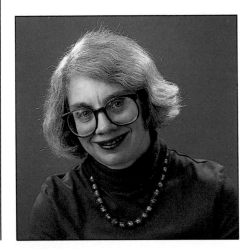

Gloria Zeche, 48

The long, weighty, one-layer hairstyle dragged down the lines of Gloria's face. The greenish charcoal shade of gray robbed her face of color. When Gloria's naturally wavy hair was layered, curl began to appear here and there. A rich red-brown color was mixed for Gloria, a little lighter and brighter than her natural color before "going gray." The color was applied, and the hair was blown dry and combed. Next the eyebrows were arched, a beige base and bright rose blusher were applied to bring color to Gloria's face, and a smoky gray and a deep purple eye shadow were used on her eyelids. Next came a black eyeliner pencil to outline the upper eyelid, then black mascara and bright pink lipstick. The makeup worked well with the glasses too. "I look so striking," she said.

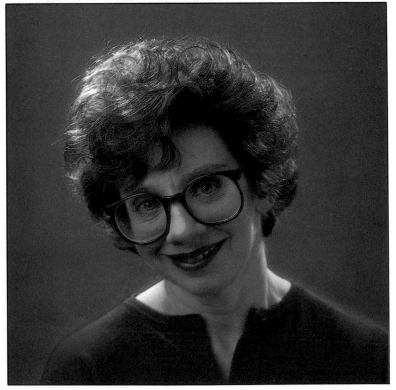

Ruth Ann Cranston, 46

The straight lines and blunt, medium-length cut were too severe for Ruth Ann's age and facial shape. For more height, softness, and shape, her hair was layered on the crown and on the sides. For a look that said Ruth Ann spent plenty of time in the sun, selected strands of hair were pulled through a cap and painted with a blond toner. Then her hair was blown dry, the sides brushed up off her face to emphasize the eyes, and the hair combed up at the top to provide volume. Several strands were combed forward, to suggest bangs. For the face a beige foundation, translucent powder, pink cheek color, neutral eye shadow with a touch of eyeliner, and black mascara. And finally bright red lipstick was applied to make the lips look fuller. "Is this really me?" asked Ruth Ann. "I love it."

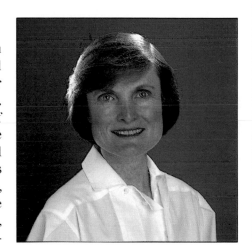

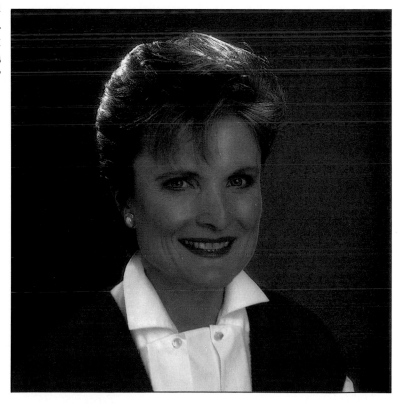

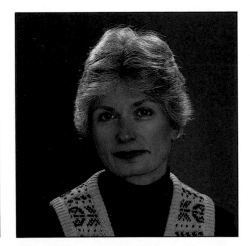

Louise Greiner, 43

The color was fine, but Louise's hairstyle was too rounded and heavy on the sides. It was cut away to flatter the eyes and cheekbones. Because gray hair becomes discolored easily, a platinum colored "glaze" was applied to Louise's hair to make it shinier. Then it was blown dry and the sides brushed back and the hair lifted at the crown for volume. Makeup was simple: a light foundation, some cheek color, a bit of eye shadow, some eyeliner and mascara, and a flattering lipstick. "I love the shine in my hair, and I love the makeup," said Louise. She was skeptical at first about the job of maintaining the hairstyle, but several days later Louise reported, "I love it now."

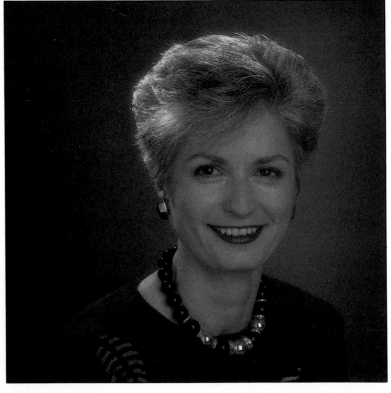

Candice's and Walter's Plan for Ruth Ann

Candice felt the straight lines and blunt medium-length cut were not flattering to Ruth Ann's face. Candice would change the shape by layering her hair. "I want to take the emphasis away from her jaw and call attention to her eye line and cheekbones," said Candice. "Her current haircut is too severe for her age and the shape of her face." She needs layering on top to give her height, shape, and softness. Candice and Walter also thought, because of the texture and color of Ruth Ann's hair, warm gold highlights all over would enhance it. "Medium brown hair like Ruth Ann's should look as if she spent a lifetime in the sun," said Candice. The variation in color would make her hair look thicker and brighter. It wouldn't camouflage her hair but would be an enhancement like makeup. Highlights shouldn't be ash colored," said Candice. "Ash is aging."

Ruth Ann After

Her Hair

After her hair was washed and towel-dried, her hair was parted on the left and layered on the crown and on the sides. Ruth Ann, who had considered her hair already short, couldn't believe the amount cut—was it too much? Before she could find out, Walter took over. To give her hair the look that said she "spent all her time in the sun," he used the cap method; that is, he pulled selected strands of hair through a cap and painted them with a blonde toner (reassuring Ruth Ann that she would not need to have a "coloring job" more than every four months). The cap method is the best way to color thin hair like Ruth Ann's. Candice blew Ruth Ann's hair dry, brushing the sides up off her face to emphasize her eyes, and combed it up at the top to give it volume. Several short strands were combed forward to suggest bangs.

Her Makeup

With her fingers, Gigi applied a simple beige water-based foundation. Then she dusted on loose translucent powder; brushed on pink cheek color to accentuate the cheekbones; and applied a neutral eye shadow, a touch of eyeliner, and black mascara to bring out Ruth Ann's blue eyes. The last step was lipstick: Gigi "overlined" Ruth Ann's lips to make them fuller and "more pointy in the center" and filled in bright red lipstick using a brush.

Ruth Ann's Reaction

"Is this really me? I love it."

LOUISE GREINER, 43 (photos, page 102) ————————————

Louise Before

Louise, the membership director of the Municipal Arts Society, a nonprofit organization, is a runner. She runs six mornings a week, getting up at 5:15 A.M. to take off for a five-mile sprint around the reservoir. Her hair was a beautiful, thick, silvery gray that she wore short. But it had been cut so that it grew out round and shapeless. She wanted a casual cut (one that looked nice even at 5:15 A.M.), but she was not doing the most with the cut she had. Louise is one of the lucky ones: After the shower, she just washes and combs it, not using the blow dryer that could dull her hair. Louise said:

> I started turning gray when I was in my late twenties. My hair's very dark. I colored it when it first turned gray. Then when I heard reports that certain hair chemicals might cause cancer, I just left it alone. I'm lucky. Because my hair is oily, the chemicals didn't take out the luster, and the color was never that shoe-polish black that I see. The colorist said she thought the gray would come in very well because of the natural color and texture—and it did. When I was growing it out, I never had a period where the gray was discolored or grew in in unattractive patches. I wore it long until I was in my early thirties. Although I had dyed it to look younger, I began to see so many young, attractive women letting their hair grow gray. Gray hair is accepted now, and the funny thing is that more men than women tell me "Don't dye your hair."

Candice's and Walter's Plan for Louise

Although Candice agreed that Louise had one of the best heads of gray hair she had ever seen, she felt it was too round and heavy on the sides. It needed a shape that would draw attention to her eyes and a rinse that would not change the color but would make it shine. "You can highlight gray hair," Candice explained. "A rinse will make gray hair thicker and shinier but won't change the basic color."

Louise After

Her Hair

Snipping away at Louise's hair, Candice remarked that "I really work with this like a sculptural medium, cutting it into different angles. I'm conscious that it's a three-dimensional shape. When you have a lot of hair by your cheekbone like Louise does, it's unflattering to the cheekbones." Gray hair is more porous so it absorbs everything—even cooking odors. It can become discolored easily. So, after the cut, Walter applied a semipermanent platinum color coating called a "glaze" to make it shinier. Unlike a rinse, the glaze would last six weeks to a few months. After the rinse, Candice blew Louise's hair dry, brushing the sides back and lifting the hair at the crown for volume. The lines of the cut drew the focus to Louise's eyes and high cheekbones.

Her Makeup

Gigi went about making up Louise as she had the other three women. As she dabbed and gently rubbed on the magical elements, she explained her philosophy of makeup and the changing styles. "In the eighties, we say 'cheek color.' Before that it was 'blush' and before that it was 'rouge,' but it's all the same thing," Gigi said. I was surprised when she told us she did the same makeup on all four women. "In fact," she said, "I can do the same makeup on 25 different women with just one tiny bit of difference on their eyes, and still they'd all look different. I'm not creating this year's 'look.' I'm trying to bring out *their* features. I use a foundation to get rid of bad skin tones, undereye cover to get rid of bags or puffs, cheek color to bring out the cheekbones, and eye shadow to bring out the eyes."

Louise's Reaction

"I love the makeup, and I love the shine in my hair, but I'm not sure about the style. I'm not sure I'll be able to do it myself. Won't it just fly out? Louise was skeptical. Candice assured her that most women are shocked by change, but several days later Candice happened to run into Louise on the street. She asked her how she liked her hair? "I love it now," said Louise.

So you see that gray can be great and made even greater. A reshaping and a rinse can make fine-textured hair look thicker.

IS GRAY GOOD FOR YOU? AND WHAT IF IT ISN'T?

You saw two gray-haired makeovers on the last few pages. In one case we kept the gray; in the other we dyed the gray to a rich, warm brown. The rule we followed was simple: Louise Greiner's gray enhanced her face; Gloria Zeche's gray, which had a greenish cast, did not.

This doesn't mean you automatically cover gray. You don't. Generally gray is a way of adjusting your hair color to match the subtle—and sometimes not so subtle—changes in facial coloration that come with aging. "To have your hair gray is often more effective than to color it," says hairstylist James Reda. Walter Chadwick, the colorist who did our four makeovers, agrees that you don't automatically change gray because it's there. "Louise's hair had more of a white cast, which is generally prettier than most grays," he said. When gray hair has a yellow or greenish cast—as in Gloria's case—or if the gray is coming in in uneven patches, you may want to consult a colorist.

But here is a warning. You must go to a *good* colorist, or you could turn out to be one of those blue-haired ladies we see so often. If your area doesn't have a good colorist, better stay with the hair color you already have and enhance it with rinses or henna.

COLOR RINSES FOR GRAY HAIR

✔ *Silver hair* that's just yellowing requires a platinum or slate rinse to get rid of the yellow.

✔ *Blonde to light brown hair* with a few patches of gray needs a blonde to dark brown rinse to give a highlighted appearance.

✔ *Medium to dark brown hair* with some gray strands needs a light to medium brown rinse.

✔ *Copper red hair* requires a strawberry blonde rinse for a highlighted effect.

✔ *Auburn hair* needs a light auburn rinse. If it starts to get an overall "pinky" look, add more gold tone to the rinse.

✔ *Black hair* with less than 20 percent gray needs a dark brown rinse.

Remember the rule: If your hair is less than 20 percent gray, go one shade lighter to keep hair from becoming flat and monotone. Hair will look shaded and avoid the shoe-polish look—one of the pitfalls of semipermanent hair color. Since there's no peroxide in a semipermanent rinse, you only change the gray, not the original color.

IF YOU DECIDE TO COLOR THE GRAY

Nothing is worse than a bad home hair dye job except getting a bad one and paying for it at a salon. The problem with home hair dyes is that they work in one process. Color comes out of the bottle and onto your head. This makes the hair all one color (shoe-polish black, harsh red or blonde, flat brown), which doesn't look like real hair. Hair is many different colors; that's what gives it highlights. Most home dye "jobs" and bad ones from salons come out looking flat. "This is what gives hair coloring a bad name," said Walter. Bad hair coloring may leave your hair dry at the ends (as Milena Krondl's was), so that it's either darker or lighter at that point. Bad hair coloring like the standard "country club" blonde streaking (the one that makes you look like a zebra, as James Reda says) always looks artificial. The idea with good hair coloring is for it to look like it grew out of your own scalp—in other words, to look real.

FINDING A GOOD COLORIST

How do you find a good colorist? Much the same way that you would find a good doctor. You ask around. You notice hair that looks particularly lovely—that has a wonderful color—and you get up the courage to ask the woman it belongs to where she had it done. Be warned, however, that if it looks that good, it might be her own natural hair color.

When you get a recommendation for a colorist, call for a consultation. There are many questions you should ask, including how often you must have it done and how much it will cost. In that connection, consider this tip: If you have your hair highlighted in a variety of browns and golds, or browns and reds, mixed with your gray (and if the basic color is not far off from the depth of your own natural color), you won't be as aware of emerging undyed hair roots between touch-ups. And the touch-ups may only be necessary every six to eight weeks.

"A good hair colorist will not have a cookie-cutter selection of colors for clients but will deal with each woman individually," said Walter. "There is no single right or wrong color for any woman—gray, in fact, may be a good color choice."

You can't give a blanket answer about gray. "Much depends on its placement, whether it comes in evenly or in patches, and whether it is a pretty shade of gray," said Walter. "When you start going gray, a little highlighting might be nice," he added. "When your hair is over 50 percent gray and the color is unbecoming, you might want to consider a color change."

NEVER GO FAR
FROM YOUR NATURAL COLOR

Generally for any color change a good colorist keeps the new color within the same depth as your original hair color. Take Milena Krondl's hair for example. Her original hair color was a medium brown. So auburn was a better color for her, as it came nearer the tone of her original hair color than the carrot shade that had developed over years of her home dying efforts. Carrot might be a better color for someone whose original hair color was light brown or ashey blonde because it would be closer to her natural skin color. In other words, skin tone must be the deciding factor.

How to Select the Hair Color Process That's Right for You

Process	Who Should Use It	How It Works	Upkeep
Temporary rinse (also called color rinse)	For first-time color users who are unsure of what color to use; works well for women who want to enrich natural color or darken hair. Since this product contains no peroxide to bleach out color, it cannot lighten. Good for women who are just turning gray; does not change texture or dry hair	Does not color hair more than one shade, but gives it tone; liquid best applied after shampooing and towel drying	Lasts only through one washing; temporary rinses can stain pillow-cases and collars; repeated use can cause a buildup of color coating that can result in dull and lusterless hair
Semi-permanent color	For women with up to 25 percent gray hair	Coats but does not penetrate hair shaft; does not contain peroxide and so does not change structure or texture of hair. Shampoo in and leave on 20 to 30 minutes. (For at-home users, foam-type products are easier to control than liquids.) Choose a color that's a shade or two lighter than your original (no gray) hair color since those lotions tend to darken a bit	Lasts for 2 to 6 weeks, depending upon how often you shampoo
Permanent color (one process)	For women who have more than 25 percent gray and for women who like a greater change of color than semipermanent color allows	A process that uses a mixture containing ammonia, peroxide and pigment and takes effect in about 1 hour; apply with brush or bottle	Remains until hair grows out and is cut off; regrowth needs to be touched up as often as every 4 to 5 weeks

Process	Who Should Use It	How It Works	Upkeep
Permanent color (double process)	For women who look best in a pale blonde shade that cannot be achieved by one process	Hair is prelightened to a pale yellow stage; shampooed; and toner with mixture of ammonia, peroxide and pigment applied	Hair must be maintained properly for optimum condition; regrowth needs touch-up every 2 to 3 weeks
Henna rinse	For brunettes, strawberry blondes, and redheads. Be especially careful if your hair is permed, if you're naturally blonde (can turn hair green!), or if your hair is partly gray (red henna on brown hair turns gray strands very red)	A natural vegetable compound that adds rich red tones to dark or brown hair; also conditions hair and gives it luster. Comes as a powder in a variety of colors; is mixed with boiling water and a conditioner. Work through hair like a shampoo; leave on 30 minutes to 1 hour, then rinse. Reacts differently on different kinds of hair, so best to have it applied by professional	Fades gradually with washing, but not as quickly as some semi-permanent coloring; reapply every 2 to 3 months
Highlighting (also called frosting, painting, streaking, or sun-bursting)	For women with dark blonde or brown hair or light brown hair beginning to gray; not meant to cover gray but to blend with gray	Process consists of using special mixture to lighten strands of hair so result will be a variety of shades. Professional colorists use plastic pull-through cap, aluminum foil wrap, or brush to apply lightener	Permanent color that lasts from 3 to 6 months; new growth doesn't show quickly

But there are other solutions to hair color that don't go as far as dying it (which involves the use of peroxide). Gloria, for example, had a semipermanent coloring, which doesn't involve peroxide and which lasts about six weeks. It gives her a chance to live with her new color for a while and to see if it agrees with her. If it does, she can elect to go with the semipermanent color forever, merely having it touched up every six weeks. If your hair is losing luster and intensity, you can go for a vegetable-based color. These are the hennas, which give hair a red cast. They work best on all shades of brown hair, *never* on gray. You redo these every two months.

MAKE YOUR OWN RINSES

Then there are the rinses. For gray hair that is yellowing, James Reda recommends Roux White Minx. And for other hair colors, there are countless rinses that have been around since our great grandmother's day that seem to soften the hair and make it shiny. Here are a few favorites that have stood the test of time:

Lemon Rinse for Oily Blonde Hair

Lemon is a good rinse for both natural and bleached blondes (with the latter, it separates hair strands, which tend to be porous and cling together). Add the strained juice of 3 lemons to 1 pint of water. Pour this through the hair several times to brighten it.

Chamomile Rinse for Blondes

Chamomile grows wild in Vermont where I have lived at various times in my life. My friend Caroline and I used to pick it to make teas for steaming our faces, and Caroline, a blonde, used it to make a rinse for her hair. This is the rinse she used: Steep ¼ cup of chamomile flowers in 1 quart of boiling water. Strain off the liquid and cool it. Use it as a final rinse to brighten blonde hair. Do not rinse it off. This herb acts as a tonic for the scalp.

Chamomile-Vinegar Rinse for Bleached Blondes

The same chamomile rinse Caroline used brightens bleached hair if 1 teaspoon of vinegar is added to restore the acid mantle, separate strands of hair, and remove the spongy, sticky feeling that often occurs when hair is bleached.

Chamomile-Henna Rinse for Light Brown Hair

Chamomile also brightens light brown hair. An addition of 1 tablespoon of henna to the Chamomile Rinse for Blondes will give this hair color red highlights.

Rosemary Rinse for Brunette Hair

Rosemary is my favorite herb for the face and hair. I like its scent too. I rinse with an infusion of rosemary made this way: Steep 2 tablespoons of rosemary in 1 pint of boiling water. Strain off the liquid. Let it stand until cold. Rinse the hair with it to fluff it up and to bring out the natural highlights. Do not rinse it out.

Cider Vinegar Rinse for Brunette Hair

Add 2 tablespoons of vinegar to 1 quart of water. Pour this through the hair several times. Rinse it out to remove any vinegar odor. This softens dark hair and gives it luster. A vinegar rinse is also good for dark hair that has been dyed since it restores the acid mantle and separates strands of hair that may be sticky and porous.

THE LONG HAIR-SHORT HAIR AT 40-PLUS DEBATE

Ever since I can remember, the debate has raged: long or short? Long hair wearers have been accused of trying to recapture their youth (unsuccessfully) while some short haircuts have been called everything from the "menopause bob" to the tidy lady-golfer look. To try and resolve the age-old problem, I consulted with a prestigious group of experts by phone, in their salons and sometimes over tea. But imagine with me please that they are all seated at a conference table with me: Jean Adams, former beauty editor of *Redbook* and now a beauty consultant; Yves Claude of the Yves Claude Salon; Ilana Harkavi, owner of Il Makiage, a hair and skin-care salon; George Michael, known as the czar of long hair; James Reda, an independent hairstylist for magazines and TV; and Candice Robins of the David Daines Hair Salon.

I asked each one these questions: If a woman over 40 wears her hair either straight or wavy to her shoulders or longer, does she look foolish? If her hair is gray and long, must she roll it up in a bun? In short, is short hair preferable after age 40?

Jean Adams: "For most women a medium length—especially if they have good hair—is the best. Automatically cutting your hair short at 40 is a mistake. For some women it's fine and it does lift the face, but depending on the shape of her face, a longer, fuller style is actually more flattering."

Yves Claude: "Long hair is not attractive for women over 40 as it accentuates any drooping facial lines. It's best to keep it soft and layered and pulled away from the temples."

Ilana Harkavi: "The most flattering hairstyle for women over 40 is layered and chin length, so the hair casts a shadow on any problems she has at the jawline."

George Michael: "To say a woman must cut her hair because she is over 40 is ridiculous. If a woman has gorgeous, thick hair, she should show it. Men don't really like short hair. Aside from that, when you are older, you actually need more hair because of the imperfections in your face. If you wear your hair longer, you are going to look younger."

James Reda: "Wearing long one-length hair when you are over 40 makes you look like an aging Barbie doll. Over-40 hair should be short and layered and lifted from the face to give softness. Look at Elizabeth Taylor and Joan Collins. Both wear their hair layered and short. Any line that comes down around the face will emphasize downward facial lines. The more you bring the line of the hairstyle upward, the less these lines will be noticed. With short hair, however, you don't want to bring attention to the face in an unappealing way. I wouldn't ever recommend a sharp geometric style, or any other severe style. And I'm not talking about those tidy, little, lady-golfer haircuts."

Candice Robins: "Long or short hair, hair must be layered to give a woman softness around the face. I think long hair for women over 40 is fine, as long as it's not one length. And if it is, a woman should wear it up if that's a style that's becoming to her. Gray hair, in particular, should never be worn one length. It looks better layered because the layers reflect light. Short haircuts can look fabulous on women over 40. But not just any short haircut. A round cut—the kind that looks like a bowl was put on a woman's head to cut it—is the worst. It doesn't flatter facial features—and yet it's the most standard haircut."

So the debate goes on. If you're looking for the definitive answer to the question of long or short, I'd say: Think about the quality of your hair instead of its length. See a good hairstylist. Together, look in the mirror at your face. Then decide which is best.

How to Find a Good Hairstylist

Ruth Ann Cranston, our third makeover (page 101), had been the victim of a coloring job that turned her hair orange a few months before Candice did her hair. If you've ever had that happen to you, you know it can take months to grow out. It's the same thing with "butchered" hair. Experiences like these can turn you off to hairstylists. Yet a really good haircut can make the difference between dowdy and being chic at 40 plus. How can you find a good hairstylist? Yves Claude of the Yves Claude Salon, New York City, recommends that you:

✔ **Ask women whose hair you like—and whose texture is similar to yours—who did their hair.**

If you'll remember, Ruth Ann, new in the city, asked *one* woman. As it turned out, that woman had short, curly hair unlike Ruth Ann's fine, straight hair.

✔ **Visit the salon first and observe the hairstylist.**

Of course, you can't make the stylist nervous by standing nearby. So get a manicure and watch from a distance. While you're watching, see if the stylist looks at the client in the mirror while cutting her hair. In other words, he views the hair as a part of the woman, not just the hair itself.

✔ **Talk with the stylist.**

Nowadays most beauty salons suggest that you come in for a consultation to get your questions answered about your hair. It you have questions, say, "You've done my friend's hair and she thinks you're awfully good. What would you recommend for me?" Be sure the stylist asks when and if you have had a permanent or hair coloring— and if so, what kind. You should also discuss how much time you're willing to devote to the upkeep of your hair. Talk over the style you want as well, and any special problems you may have experienced with your hair in the past. Find out about record keeping. (Many fine salons make detailed dossiers of their clients' experiences with various chemical treatments.)

MORE ON WASHING, CONDITIONING, AND DRYING YOUR HAIR (AND SOME HOMEMADE HAIR REMEDIES)

How will you choose one shampoo from the drugstore's dizzying display of hair products? Inexpensive? Expensive? For oily hair? For dry hair? Protein added? Thick or thin? Scented? Balanced for pH? For babies? A shampoo with built-in conditioner? *None* of that matters, according to Candice Robins. Most women's hair suffers from product overkill. They buy according to fragrance, which is unimportant. The purpose of a shampoo is only to clean your hair thoroughly.

✔ **Make sure the hairstylist who gives you the consultation looks at you before you put on a smock or robe.**

He should observe the clothes you are wearing, your height, your makeup, and the texture of your hair—the kind of life-style you reflect. Don't wear jeans, for example, if this is not your customary attire.

If you follow this advice, you shouldn't be intimidated by the hairstylist you pick. You will be in control.

Working with Your Hairstylist

Spend money on a good haircut and advice, but do some research yourself. Read a few women's magazines. Cut out pictures of hairstyles you like. Discuss them with your hairstylist. Share in the decision about what is to be done to your hair. Don't leave it up to the stylist alone to figure out. Be open to the latest style, with variations that work for you. But don't be talked into an extreme style and sharp lines or an overly romantic, too-young hairstyle that doesn't flatter you.

There are many ways to give your hair body and shape. Most salons will share their secrets with you because they want you to know how to "do" your hair between visits. Ask about their techniques—about using mousses and gels, how to brush and comb your hair. Ask if you need a mild body wave to keep your hair under control.

If you have your hair done and you aren't pleased or don't know how to work with it once you get home, call the stylist and tell him. "A good stylist will show you how to work with the style without charging more money," says Candice Robins. "I for one don't want women walking around town looking all wrong in my hairstyles."

The fewer additives like "protein" and "placenta," the better. Thicker shampoos are not necessarily stronger than the thinner ones; in fact, thinner ones are often more concentrated. Many of us still think "protein" is magic. Forget it.

WASHING YOUR HAIR

The only purpose of a shampoo is to clean the hair and scalp. Commercial shampoos contain detergents, mild cleansers that remove oil and dirt. To be sure of mildness, Candice Robins recommends a good quality *castile* shampoo available at a natural foods store or beauty-supply store. In any case, all shampoos should be diluted 50 percent with distilled water. (Philip Kingsley says some shampoos work best if you add nine parts water to one part shampoo.) "There's a difference in product quality," advises Candice. "Learn to read labels," she urges. "Don't be seduced by additives or fragrances. The simpler the shampoo, the better." Candice recommends any Aubrey Organics Shampoo. If you can't find it locally, write to Aubrey Organics, 4419 North Manhattan Avenue, Tampa, FL 33614, and ask for a local source.

Whatever product you choose, shampooing the wrong way can do a lot of damage to your hair. Most women pour shampoo directly on their heads, rub vigorously to a lather, and then rinse. After the rinse, they pour more shampoo on, vigorously rub, then rinse again. Then they give their hair a rough towel-rub. All wrong.

THE RIGHT WAY TO SHAMPOO

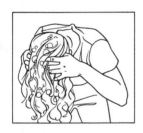

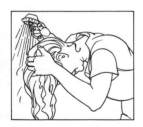

Philip Kingsley and Candice Robins agree on the proper method of shampooing: First, soak your hair. A thoroughly wet head won't require as much soap to work up a lather. Pour a small amount of diluted shampoo into the palm of your hand, rub both hands together; then, smooth the lather over your hair with the palm of your hands. Then massage your head (kneading the scalp and drawing your fingers through your hair to the ends). Don't scrub vigorously because you'll irritate your scalp. Rinse well. Shampoo left on the scalp can irritate the scalp. Rinse again. Philip Kingsley advises shampooing every day. He says, "You wash your face every day and you take your hair to the same places you take your face." But Candice says: "Wash your hair when it feels and looks dirty." Mine feels dirty every day.

If your shampoo seems to be less effective than before, it means that your hair has changed in some way. Either you've permed or bleached or tinted or sprayed your hair, or your hair reflects a physiological or environmental change. "It doesn't mean that your hair has built up a resistance to that shampoo," said Mr. Kingsley.

And while you're shampooing, don't forget the ten-minute massage advised by Mr. Kingsley. Massage by kneading the scalp; that is, move the scalp on the bone. Don't just rub. "A tight scalp indicates poor circulation, a problem common in older women," added Candice. "Good circulation, partly the result of scalp massage and exercise, stimulates hair growth. A good head of hair comes from a really good scalp." (Both Mr. Kingsley and Candice believe in taking vitamins, especially the B vitamins. Candice says she's been stirring brewer's yeast (rich in B vitamins) into her orange juice since college.

CONDITIONING YOUR HAIR

"I think women tend to use conditioners too often and incorrectly," says Candice. A conditioner is an emulsified oil (since oil and water don't mix naturally, manufacturers put in an emulsifier to distribute oil throughout the hair), and it leaves a film on the hair shaft. Too much conditioner, which never needs to go on the scalp, makes the hair flat. Conditioners are sometimes used effectively on damaged hair—hair that's been overprocessed—or long hair. I prefer to use a brilliantine. If you use a conditioner, pour a small amount of an easy-running liquid type into your palm and rub your hands together. Then apply the conditioner to your hair. Rinse.

Candice adds that all conditioners work better with heat. Caps and heating units similar to the kind used in hair salons are sold at beauty-supply stores for under $25.

It is a misconception that a conditioner makes hair shiny. Your hair grows out of your head shiny. It's true that the oil in a conditioner lets the comb go through your hair more easily, but if you are patient when combing your hair, you won't need a conditioner very often.

HOMEMADE TREATMENTS

Candice thinks the old solutions are best for hair: set with beer, club soda, or liquid gelatin; or use a high-quality castile soap as a shampoo. Here are two soap recipes and some homemade conditioners and rinses to try.

Mint Dandruff Tonic

Add 1 cup of mint leaves (fresh if available) to 1 cup of white vinegar and 2 cups of water. Boil this together slowly for 5 to 10 minutes. Strain it. Cool liquid. Before wetting your hair, rub the solution into the scalp and leave on for 2 to 4 minutes. Rinse well, then shampoo.

Egg White-Lemon Dry Scalp Treatment

Whip up the whites of 2 eggs with the strained juice of 2 lemons. Before wetting your hair, rub the mixture lavishly into the scalp with your fingertips to remove flaky, itchy residue and restore the natural oils. Leave on for 2 to 4 minutes. Rinse well, then shampoo.

Yogurt-Lemon Rind Bleached Hair Conditioner

Combine equal amounts of yogurt and grated lemon rind (1 teaspoon each for shorter hair, more for longer). Before wetting your hair, generously rub this into the scalp, pulling it through the hair. The yogurt conditions dry, sun- or chemical-bleached hair; the lemon rind adds natural oils and luster. Leave on for 2 to 4 minutes. Rinse well, then shampoo.

Egg Yolk-Yogurt Conditioner for Dull, Brittle Hair

Beat 1 egg yolk until fluffy. To it add ½ cup of yogurt and beat again until thoroughly mixed. Comb this mixture through clean hair. Leave it on for 10 minutes; then rinse thoroughly with warm water. Follow up with a vinegar rinse of ¼ cup of vinegar to 1 cup of water, and more warm water. This leaves the hair soft and lustrous.

DRYING YOUR HAIR

Let your hair dry in the air, if possible, rubbing each strand with your fingers to help the process. Don't use a brush until your hair is completely dry, as wet strands are more susceptible to breakage.

Letting your hair dry naturally is rarely practical, due to the time required. Sometimes you have to compromise. The obvious alternative is to blow hair dry. "It's not the hair dryer that's to blame for robbing the hair of moisture but how we use it," says Philip Kingsley. "You can have the best of both worlds—a quick blow-dry and soft, manageable hair." It's going from damp to dry that the potential damage is done. But even that's OK so long as you stop as soon as it's dry. If you keep the dryer on for another ten extra seconds or so, that's when the trouble starts. And when you're drying, use the lowest possible warm setting, or even cool. It may take you longer to dry your hair this way, but the extra time is worth it for the health of your hair.

If your hair is curly, don't blow-dry and don't vigorously towel-dry. (Curly hair becomes frizzy from overprocessing—bad "dye jobs"—and vigorous towel-drying.) "You should be able to get out of the shower, wrap a towel around your head for a minute or two to absorb some moisture, then let your hair dry by just running your fingers through it," advises Candice. "The less you do with it the better."

So your hair—whatever its texture or style—like your skin is a mirror of your health. There's no such thing as "bad hair." If your hair's dry and lifeless or frizzy, it reflects the overuse of hair care products or poor health. "When women take care of their health and use good products, their hair usually reflects that care," says Candice.

So you see that gray can be great and made even greater. A reshaping and a rinse can make fine hair look thicker. To combine the philosophy of my grandmother, Aunt Dorothy, and Candice: You're only as good as your hair, your hairdresser—and a good pair of shoes. With all three (or maybe just a good head of hair), you'll have the best you there is. And as the old song says, "Who Could Ask for Anything More?"

Chapter 5

MAKING YOUR OWN FACE MORE FABULOUS

Nothing tells our age more than outdated makeup: heavy eyeliner, heavily penciled eyebrows, or plum-colored lipstick. Although the rule of thumb is to keep in touch with current makeup trends, modifying them a bit if we're over 40, a lot of us cling to the looks that were in style when we were in our teens or early twenties. We're caught in the past and that makes us look old.

As for my past, I first became aware of the power of cosmetics as a ten-year old when I left California to visit Uncle Ned and Aunt Dorothy and their five daughters in New York. I remember the serious application of glossy red lipstick to produce Hollywood-starlet mouths, lipstick smears on napkins and glasses, and the click of compacts snapping shut (often in unison) if two cousins were present. Their mother, my Aunt Dorothy, was a "career woman" (who fancied herself as a Ginger Rogers look-alike) and seized upon each new makeup style as it came along.

Since the late 1930s, she had been wearing Max Factor's Pan-Cake, a water-soluble cake foundation, and you could see the obvious line between Aunt Dorothy's face and neck. She had drawers full of cosmetics, including mascara, which she moistened by spitting discreetly on the dark little cake. Hollywood, of course, set the makeup fashions. Aunt Dorothy was one of the few "ordinary women" who wore eye makeup (iridescent eye shadow in emerald, sapphire, amethyst, or turquoise) and collected ads for contour cream, crow's-foot cream, deep pore cleanser, pore pastes, and the like. She said she would need them someday, "and Donna, so will you."

I thought she was crazy. Me! I couldn't imagine being older than 12. I was fascinated, even at that age, by "leg makeup," a soupy brown lotion created to replace nylons when they were unavailable during World War II. My 19-year-old cousin Martha's predate ritual included the application of "leg makeup," and I worried with her that it would ruin her clothes by rubbing off on them.

The drawers and dressing tables in this family of women (oh, poor Uncle Ned!) were filled with lipsticks in colors called Dangerous Red, Pixie Pink, Cherries in the Snow, Stop Red, and Sky Blue Pink. Martha even went through a phase of gluing beauty marks on her face—a fad that lasted only a short time. She thought she looked like Lana Turner and hoped everyone else would think so, too. A few years later, Martha went in for what *Vogue* called "the doe-eyed look," a look that involved eye shadows, eyebrow pencils, mascara, and eye liner in an obvious inky line that encircled her eyes and tapered into Bambi-like points on the outer edges. During one period, Martha wore one color of lipstick on the bottom lip and another on the top. Martha "rouged" her cheeks and told me how lucky we were: Our great grandmothers, she knew, had to rub a moistened red ribbon on their faces to redden their cheeks. Martha, a very plain girl, tried for the "glamour girl" look and modeled herself after movie stars like Loretta Young and Joan Crawford.

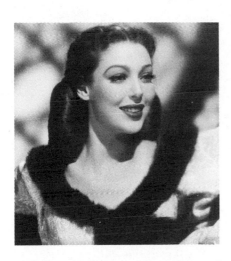
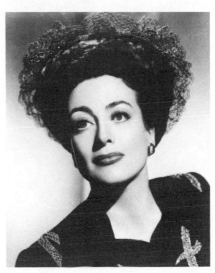

I thought all this was terribly adult. One day I, too, would have a scarlet mouth and inky eyes. Alas, this was not to be. In my teens, the "natural look" was born. One strived to look like the girl next door. My heroines (and those of my peers) were Doris Day and Jane Powell—preferably we all wanted to look like California blondes with snub noses and perky personalities.

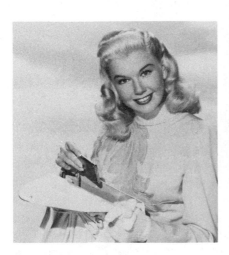
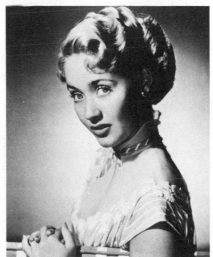

The point of all this is that for as long as I can remember, women have believed makeup was useful for trying to look like somebody else. It never occurred to us that we could and should look like ourselves. Even while we feigned a "natural look," it was someone else's natural good looks we were after. Well, here's a surprise. Makeup is useful for bringing out the best of nobody else but you.

Makeup Tools—The Basics

Applying your makeup with the proper tools is essential. After you experiment, you may want to subtract from or add to this basic list.

Face
Cotton swabs
Latex sponges
Several sable
  brushes for
  powder and
  blusher
Sterile absorbent
  cotton balls

Lips
Lip brush
Lip pencil

Eyes
Eyebrow brush
Eyelash curler
Magnifying mirror
Sharpener for eye
  pencils
Tweezers (available
  with pointed,
  slanted, or
  straight tip—
  you'll find which
  type works best
  for you)

40-PLUS MAKEUP TIPS FROM THE EXPERTS

When the opportunity came, I took full advantage of it by asking a group of makeup experts for basic tips we can all use.

SEVEN GOOD POINTS FROM PEGGY ESPOSITO

At 27, Peggy is a Gina Lollobrigida look-alike who doesn't worry about growing older. She believes your looks should be an expression of who you are. For example, don't try to look like Christie Brinkley if your looks are more like Barbara Streisand's (who's no frump and is closer to your age). If your hair is curly, don't take an iron to it (as young women did in the sixties). If you're 40 or 50 or 60, emphasize the best points about you at that age. Don't try to change yourself into somebody else. Look like the best part of *you.*

Among the worst mistakes women over 40 can make are these: wearing severe, sharply defined eyeliner, harsh rouge or blusher, lipstick that is too dark, and contour that is not blended properly. And heavy, tinted face powder is definitely all wrong. Always use transparent powder.

To contour the cheekbones, apply contour cream below the most prominent part of your cheekbone. Blusher goes on the bone and not too near the nose.

Shy away from frosted eye colors except for evening. If a woman moves in a high-fashion milieu and dresses accordingly with glamorous jewelry, she might bend the rule. Still, if she has crepey, drooping eyelids, it's not a good idea.

To apply eye shadow, use a sponge-tip applicator. One end is pointy and the other is not. For the most natural look, use several colors of eye shadow blended very carefully.

For retouching makeup during the day, carry a compact of translucent powder. Lancôme's Macquifinish is a good one. If your face starts to get shiny, blot it on with a powder puff. Carry cotton swabs for doing touchups under the eyes if eyeliner runs. It seems that lipstick always needs to be retouched. Eye makeup lasts longer. If you're going out after work, you may have to darken your blush to accommodate dimmer lighting.

To make your lipstick last longer, first apply a lip-color base, such as Lipfix by Elizabeth Arden. The more moist your lips are, the less lipstick they will absorb. Dab a little moisturizer on the outer part of your lips as well. After that, brush on translucent powder. Outline lips with a pencil to keep the lipstick from feathering. Then apply your lipstick.

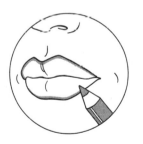

To disguise neck creases, wear scarves—especially during the daytime. If you like to use a lot of jewelry, wear a high-neck blouse with several strands of pearls as well. For evening, a choker is glamorous.

MANY POINTS FROM JAMES REDA

James, a makeup artist for personalities appearing on TV and in magazines, is in his forties. A kind, gentle, erudite man with slightly graying hair, he is given to reading philosophy. I've known him for years and count him among the people I admire. He has a fine character and believes that inner beauty beats any makeup.

Skin may become sallow as a woman gets older, and this calls for a lighter shade of foundation, one with a pink or peach tone in it.

To minimize the creases, wrinkles, and open pores that often accompany aging, wear a lighter water-based foundation that can be

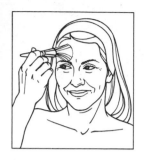

made even lighter by adding a spray of mineral water to a dime-size drop of base. Heavier foundation will seep into creases and lines on the face and will emphasize them. Apply with a moist sponge so it evens out on the skin. Blend the foundation into the neck. Instead of using a heavy pressed powder, use loose, fine translucent powder and apply gently with a large sable brush.

To conceal age spots and broken vessels, cover them with Madeleine Mono light undereye concealer. Apply it with a short, stiff brush so it doesn't cake.

To camouflage a double chin, apply a shade of foundation that is one to two shades darker than you are wearing on your face and blend carefully so there will not be a line. Brush powder on over it to help soften any line.

To avoid makeup seepage, use a powder blusher instead of a cream, which is too thick, too bright, and seeps into the pores.

To minimize crepiness and creases of the eyelids, avoid using cream eye shadow, which emphasizes these problems. Use a powder eye shadow, instead, in charcoals, grays, and tawny peach tones that brighten your eyes.

To open up the eyes, use the same color for eye shadow that you use for blusher when appropriate. Peach, for example, will open the eyes wider. You can also wear a peach tone on the brow bone.

To avoid a dated look, never wear bright blue or green eye shadow; they make your eyes look like two stoplights. Shadow should be blended up and outward. Never wear false eyelashes. Only a minimal amount of makeup should be applied on the eyelids of a woman who is past 50.

To get rid of bagginess under the eyes, apply cold compresses, such as cotton balls soaked in ice water. A concealer won't cover up puffiness and may even emphasize it.

To prevent lip color from bleeding into tiny whistle lines around your mouth, don't wear gloss with lipstick.

If you want to de-emphasize yellowing teeth, don't wear orange lipstick.

TWO BIG POINTS FROM LIA SCHORR

At 40 she is the director of Lia Schorr Skin Care, New York. She grew up on a kibbutz and was a soldier in the Israeli army. The best time of her life is now, she says. One reason is that Lia has an adorable year-old daughter who spends her days with her mom at the office. Lia is a skin specialist and makeup stylist, but she feels that no amount of powder, shadow, and greasepaint can compensate for skin that is not at its best. "There is nothing like health and happiness for good skin—that and romance."

For glowing skin at any age, get lots of sleep. Always remove your makeup before you exercise or go to sleep. Avoid spicy, fried, and sweet food, coffee, smoking, and excessive alcohol, all of which can bring a dullness to the skin that even makeup can't hide. Cut out your bad habits of the past, such as keeping late hours and partying. And at all costs avoid excessively tinted or heavily scented makeup.

To set makeup and make it last, first apply eye cream and moisturizer. Put small dabs of concealing cream all around the eyes with a small sponge. This also acts as an eye shadow base. With a sponge, apply a thin film of foundation over your face and throat. Dust loose transparent powder all over your face with a large brush. Then apply eye and cheek color. Finish by dusting more of the powder over your face again. Set makeup by spraying a fine mist of water over your face.

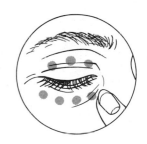

FIVE TERRIFIC POINTS FROM GIGI WILLIAMS

Gigi, 39, a makeup stylist for television, screen, and magazines thinks women need not worry so much about applying makeup. It's really not such a big deal, she says.

To gain confidence about makeup, take one professional makeup lesson; it is well worth the expense. You'll learn how to apply makeup and shape eyebrows to give your eyes a lift instead of pulling them down. Practice. Then, when you know the procedure really well, you should be able to apply your makeup in minutes.

The Proper Lighting for Applying Makeup

Ideally, makeup should be applied in natural lighting—preferably a bright north light mainly by a window. Most bathroom lights give a distorted impression. Office lighting can make women look yellow and green, but you can't do much about it. And it's absurd to think that you can make up especially for work just because the lighting there is unflattering! The big difference in lighting is between the day and evening. The general rule is that you intensify color in the evening —make it brighter, stronger, and even glittery.

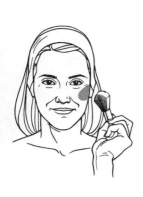

To make lipstick last, try dime-store lipsticks. Some last longer than expensive department-store lipsticks because they're drier. They contain stains that adhere better and longer without irritating the lips the way color dyes did years ago. In fact, one amazing lipstick, Liplife, is colorless when you apply it. Then, depending on your chemistry, it turns red or pink within 20 minutes and stays on until you wash it off.

To make foundation last all day, apply foundation in downward strokes with your fingers. Fingers are gentler and have more control that a sponge. When you stroke *down* (rather than in a circular motion), you do a better job of covering your pores and protecting your skin from the elements.

For thicker lashes use black mascara instead of brown, and apply one coat instead of two. Less is always better.

To apply cheek color, put it *only* on the *outside* part of cheek (from a point that would coincide with the outer rim of the iris if you were to draw a line from there down to your cheekbone). Apply only on the cheekbone, smoothing the color up into your temple.

FIVE FABULOUS MAKEOVERS

Here you have five amazing makeovers performed by two makeup artists, Peggy Esposito and James Reda, who create makeup for people who appear on television and on magazine covers. Peggy Esposito did the first five makeovers. James Reda did the makeover for our Ford model who wanted an updated look. Now you will see that each woman who participated in the makeovers—women like you and I—all turned out to be stunning or at least better-looking versions of their own very special selves.

JEANNE CONLON, 44 (photos, page 135) ─────────────

Jeanne Before

Jeanne, married to an artist and the mother of a 12-year-old son, is a photographer's and stylist's representative. When Jeanne arrived at the studio for her makeover, she wore jeans and a preppy alligator T-shirt. She likes clothes by Laura Ashley and L. L. Bean. Her hair, streaked blonde and curled in a flip, had been recently styled but needed coloring at the roots. Jeanne said:

> I don't wear makeup base because makeup was unfashionable when
> I was young in the preppy-look era of the early sixties. I do wear

undereye concealer and a little blusher. I've always tried to de-emphasize my large nose (snub noses were in style in the sixties) and my southern Italian looks and have gone for the perky, blonde look as much as I could. I hope Peggy can tell me how to conceal these dark spots that appeared on my face during my pregnancy. I absolutely don't want any major changes. I have kinky, curly hair, which I've blown straight with a dryer for 20 years. Aside from that I have it streaked regularly, which makes it even drier, and the blower adds to the dryness. I've worn this style since I was a freshman in college. I'm too conservative to change.

Peggy's Plan for Jeanne

Peggy took issue with what Jeanne said, telling her that she needed a trendier, more dramatic look in both her makeup and her clothes—something that looked southern Italian, which Jeanne was after all. She said she could cover Jeanne's "pregnancy spots" and the dark circles under her eyes. But she also said she would play up the best of Jeanne's ethnic features—her "aristocratic" nose and her good, strong mouth, while she would minimize the downward lines of her eyes and eyebrows.

"Jeanne's eyes are deeply set," said Peggy, so she would shadow and shade her eyes upward. She would minimize her down lines. She would make Jeanne's face look broader through the cheek area and would minimize her broad jawline. She wouldn't change the shape of her mouth, but said that Jeanne *should* wear lipstick. "She needs more than gloss to brighten her face," said Peggy. The lines of her haircut were too harsh for her face and her nose. Jeanne's hair hanging down pulled all the features of her face downward. The hair should be brought up to emphasize her eyes and bring out her very interesting profile.

Finally, Peggy felt that Jeanne's clothes were too collegiate and that a sophisticated European look would be more flattering. She's tall and thin—and worked as a photographer's and stylist's rep—so she could carry off trendy clothes.

Jeanne After

Her Skin

A special base concealer (Lydia O'Leary's Covermark) was applied to cover the dark circles under her eyes and the "pregnancy spots" at various points on her face. After putting a moisturizer on her face, a peach-tone foundation was applied with a small foam sponge to her forehead, cheeks, chin, and nose to cover her sallow complexion. Next, translucent powder was dusted on with a large sable brush.

Her Cheeks

A brownish contour shading was gently brushed underneath the bone and blended carefully to emphasize her cheekbones. (That also draws attention to the eyes.) After the contour, a mauve powder blusher to brighten her sallow complexion was dusted on the "ball" of Jeanne's cheek and blended using circular strokes.

Her Nose

Shading was applied just under the tip and down the sides to "slim" her nose, as it is slightly broad.

Her Eyes

A light brown shadow was applied to the lids to bring out her deep-set lids, and a warm brown shadow was put on the brow bone area to diminish the puffiness around her eyes. A charcoal brown eyeliner pencil was used to draw a line from the middle of the top lid to the midway spot just below her lower lids. This line was carefully blended with a sponge-tip applicator.

Her Lips

A lip pencil in a color slightly darker than her mauve lipstick was used to outline her lips. This was filled in with the mauve lipstick to give her face color.

Her Hair

The sides were brushed up and fastened with a clip. She pushed the rest of her hair back into a fastener. This also helped to de-emphasize Jeanne's nose and accentuate her eyes. And for a touch of drama, she was given one great-looking earring and a silver gray Italian silk shirt to wear.

Jeanne's Reaction

"I really *love* this look; I just hope my husband and son will approve. I'm not sure they'll recognize me."

SUE NIRENBERG, 50 (photos, page 136)

Sue Before

Sue, divorced and the mother of three grown children, is a writer. Unlike Jeanne, she wanted "as much done as possible." Her face needed color. Her eyebrows were too dark for her hair color, and they obviously needed shaping. Her hair was in a "nonstyle"—the result of a bad permanent that was in the process of growing out. And she arrived wearing a V-neck khaki wool sweater that revealed deep creases in her neck. Sue said:

> Until about a year ago, I thought I was still in my thirties, so I wore the same makeup I had always worn. In the last year I've been horrified to notice that I have jowls and that the creases in my neck get deeper by the day. I also hate the tiny lines around my mouth; my lipstick runs in them after a few hours. When I look in the mirror, I think, "Who is that dowdy person?" Since I began working at home, I've paid less attention to my hair and clothes. Oh, please make me look like Joan Collins!

Peggy's Plan for Sue

Sue wanted to look glamorous, not dowdy. Whether she would end up looking like Joan Collins was rather speculative. But she could look like a more terrific Sue. First, she was wearing lipstick that was too dark—a habit carried over from the forties when she first began to use lipstick. Her complexion needed brightening with the right shade of base and blusher. Her eyebrows needed plucking and shaping to minimize the downward lines on her face. Also the contrast of the dark eyebrows against Sue's face and hair was too sharp, making her look older than she was. Her jowls also made her look older. But Peggy felt she could diminish them by giving Sue a firmer-looking jawline through contouring and a more uplifting hairstyle.

Sue After

Her Skin

To hide the discoloration under Sue's eyes, Peggy applied a beige shade of Covermark with a hint of pink to perk up her pale complexion. After moisturizing, a dot of light-textured base in a light pink was applied to Sue's face, using a foam-rubber sponge. Then loose translucent powder was dusted on using a large sable brush.

Her Cheeks

To give a rosy glow to her complexion, a pinkish coral powdered blusher was applied to the ball of her cheeks and the tip of her nose and blended using circular strokes.

To give her jawline a stronger line and minimize her jowls, a soft brown contour powder was applied *underneath* the jawline with a brush.

To create a more dramatic bone structure, the same contour powder was applied with a brush at the temples and right on the brow bone.

Her Eyes

Peggy tweezed the ends of Sue's eyebrows to create an upward line. To bring out the blue of her eyes, teal eyeliner was applied on the lid next to the lashes and a peach shadow put on the brow bone. To make the eyes appear larger, the lashes were curled with an eyelash curler that was warmed in hot tap water to help hold the curl. Because her lashes were pale, black mascara (which appears brown over pale lashes) was applied to the upper lashes to make them look thicker and longer.

Her Lips

Her lips were outlined with a coral pencil liner and filled in with a coral lipstick.

Her Hair

The hair around her face was layered to create more volume and height and to give some uplift to her face.

Sue's Reaction

"I can't believe it's me. Wow, what a difference. I vow I will take the time every day to do this. Once you know how much better you can look, it seems worth the extra effort to keep it up. I may never have the sultry looks I've always envied, but I certainly don't look dowdy anymore. I may not look like Joan Collins, but I look like a pretty Sue, don't I?"

ABIGAIL THOMAS, 44 (photos, page 137) ————————————————

Abigail Before

When Abigail Thomas, an editor and a mother of four grown children (and a grandmother of two), arrived at the studio for her makeover, she looked pale and tired. Her hair, which is the color of her skin, was pinned up in a "mop" style. She was trying to compensate for her pale skin and a hair color that matched it by wearing bright clothes instead of using makeup. Although she wore a dab of purplish lipstick, the purples and pinks she was wearing were the wrong colors. Instead of enhancing her skin tones, they drained her color. Abigail said:

> I've never really learned how to select or apply makeup. If I knew how to apply it, I would wear it. I'd like a soft, natural look I can wear everyday—one that's easy for me to do. If I can come away from this makeover with one small essential thing I've learned about makeup—one small thing that will make a change in the way I look—this will have been a successful experience.

Peggy's Plan for Abigail

Abigail had no skin problems. In fact, she had lovely skin. She just wasn't making much effort to look her best. Peggy planned to enhance Abigail's prominent nose and good cheekbones with contour. Like Jeanne, Abigail's hanging-down, shapeless hair locked her into the look she had (and could get away with) in her twenties. It was too long, too wild, and out of control. But it was great hair—with a thick texture and a pretty honey color. It simply needed reshaping. Her clothes were "vintage hippie"—loose, casual, outdated. She needed warmer tones in her clothes and makeup—rust, apricot, gold, coral, rather than the cool lavenders and pinks she wore.

Abigail After

Her Skin

To conceal the dark circles under her eyes, Covermark concealer was applied. After moisturizer, a soft, light-textured, peach-tone base was put on with a foam-rubber sponge. Then, loose translucent powder was applied with a large sable brush.

Her Cheeks

To bring out the peach tones in Abigail's complexion, a powdered peach blusher was applied to her cheeks. To emphasize her prominent cheekbones, taupe contour powder was brushed on under her cheekbones.

Her Nose

To make her nose appear narrower, taupe contour powder was also applied to the sides and to the tip.

Her Eyes

With a small sponge applicator, light brown shadow was applied to her eyelids. Then to emphasize the gold in her hair and the gold tones of her skin, a slight hint of gold highlighting was swept from the inner to the outer edge of the eyelid up to the brow bone. Her eyebrows were filled in with sharp, medium brown pencil strokes. Her lashes were curled with an eyelash curler, again warmed in hot top water. Because Abigail's lashes were already dark, a light brown mascara was applied.

Her Lips

Terra-cotta lip liner was used to outline them. They were filled in with a terra-cotta lipstick.

Her Hair

It was "tamed" by cutting it into soft layers to shoulder length.

Abigail's Reaction

"I wouldn't have believed that my looks could change so much. My daughter is sure to say that I could get a part on 'Dynasty.'"

ELGA STULMAN, 53 (photos, page 138) ───────────────────

Elga Before

Elga Stulman, married and the mother of four children, is an educational social worker. She runs four miles every day. She said she wanted makeup advice because her skin tone had changed and her facial lines seemed more noticeable lately. Elga said:

> I wonder if I should be using the makeup I've always used. My skin has an olive cast to it—shades of my Polish-Russian ancestry—and it has never bothered me before. But now I think my skin could use some pinkish tones, and I'd like to disguise the creases around my mouth and neck, if possible. I like the color of my hair, and in general I'm pleased with my looks.

Peggy's Plan for Elga

Peggy agreed that Elga needed brighter makeup not only because of her olive complexion but because she wears a lot of black clothes. The few neck creases were not a serious problem. Peggy thought Elga's bangs were too long; they concealed her forehead and the upper part of her eyes. "Lifting" them with a comb revealed her eyes, and makeup would make them look larger. She also intended to brighten Elga's dark olive complexion and sharpen her features.

Elga After

Her Skin

To conceal the dark circles under her eyes, Covermark concealer was applied. After applying moisturizer, a pink-tone cream base was applied to her forehead, cheeks, and chin with a small foam wedge, then carefully blended with fingertips. Then translucent powder was applied over her face with a large sable brush.

Her Cheeks

To brighten her dark olive complexion, a loose mauve powder blusher was dusted on. To "slim" Elga's slightly broad nose, a pink-tone contour was applied down the sides with a brush. The same shade of contour was used under the cheekbones.

Her Eyes

Her brow bone was shaded with brownish plum powder. A light pink powder was used just under the brow. A light gray eye shadow was applied upward at the corner of the eye to make her eyes stand out. Brown pencil was applied at the eyebrow in short feather strokes. Her lashes were curled with an eyelash curler, again warmed in hot water. Dark brown mascara was applied to her upper lashes.

Her Lips

A bright red pencil was used to outline them. Then they were filled in with a bright red lipstick to add to her new, brighter look.

Her Hair

To give Elga a more contemporary look, the bangs were lifted off her face.

Elga's Reaction

"I look a whole lot healthier now. I thought running four miles a day was enough to make me look healthy, but cosmetics have helped me to look even better."

LIZ ATWOOD, 46 (photos, page 139) ─────────────────────────

Liz Before

Liz wanted some makeup tips now that she was noticing some signs of growing older—mostly laugh lines around the mouth, tiny "whistle" lines over her lips, and darker circles under her eyes. She wasn't sure if she was making herself up properly—was her lipstick too bright for her age? Was she wearing subtle enough colors?

> I don't want to look too bright. I think that when a woman is 40 plus, her makeup should look—well—believable. I want a healthy, fresh look—not a made-up look. My skin also seems a bit drier now than it used to be. There is no apparent reason for that. I've been using moisturizer and a glycerine soap twice a day since I was 22.

James's Plan for Liz

James thought Liz needed to minimize the lines that bothered her. He would use a makeup style he considered particularly effective for women in their forties, one that would give Liz a healthy, fresh look.

Her Skin

First moisturizer was applied with a small sponge to make Liz's skin look less dry. Next, a peach-tone cream concealer was applied under the eyes to minimize her dark circles. Using a sponge, a water-based peach-tone foundation (which is less likely to clog pores than an oil-based one he might use for a younger woman) was applied to her forehead, nose, chin, and cheeks, and smoothed into her skin. Finally, a loose translucent powder was applied with a large sable brush.

Her Cheeks

To add color, James used a powder blusher in peach instead of a cream blusher, because cream collects in the open pores, which are more common in women past 40.

Her Eyes

To make Liz's eyes look more open, her eyelashes were curled. To thicken the upper lashes, a dark brown mascara was applied. To give a soft look to the eye, a blend of plum, taupe, and charcoal powdered eye shadow was applied all over the lid with a sponge-tip applicator.

Her Lips

A coral lip-liner pencil was used to outline them. Then a coral lipstick was applied.

Her Hair

Liz's hair was set with hot rollers and brushed away from her face.

Liz's Reaction

"I think it's important to realize that your face changes gradually even though you may not notice it right away. I think James has given me some pointers on how to achieve a more natural look—I like it."

USING MAKEUP TO MINIMIZE FACIAL FLAWS

Try to look as pretty as you can. Don't worry about looking chic or whether your eye shadow is the latest "in" color. If it looks great on, wear it. (Of course, you still want to look as up-to-date as possible.) Pretty usually means a softer, natural color for lipstick or blusher: mauve, pink, or rose; for eye shadow: blue, green, or plum. Extremely vivid or unusual colors may call attention to a facial flaw.

FIRST, THE BASICS

Don't be afraid to use makeup to brighten your face. You can carry off more than you think.

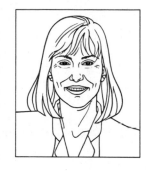

Use the right hairstyle to help hide or detract from facial flaws. Soft bangs, for example, cover up forehead lines. And styles that softly brush forward onto your cheekbones camouflage scarring or acne pitting that extends up into the hairline. Like any special feature, healthy, beautiful, shiny hair in an attractive style helps draw the focus away from problem areas elsewhere.

Apply a matte finish on troubled skin; it looks better than a shiny one. Shiny makeup reflects light and emphasizes blemished areas. Also avoid moisturizers that add shine. Get a matte finish by dusting translucent powder over makeup. Blot off excess with a folded, damp paper towel. And carry tissues with you to remove excess oil and perspiration during the day.

Be sure to remove corrective makeup thoroughly and gently, since it is often necessary to wear more of it. Albolene cream is a good, inexpensive cleanser that quickly cuts through heavy makeup. Follow cleansing with an astringent (if your skin is normal or oily), or a freshener (if your skin is normal-to-dry) to remove any residual cleanser.

Consult a well-informed salesperson when you buy new makeup, particularly a corrective one. He or she can help you choose the right color and show you how to blend it. Nine out of ten times women come home with the wrong shade only because they didn't ask for help.

SKIN

Want to cover a pimple or a temporary blemish? Pat foundation or cover-up cream in a shade slightly lighter than your complexion directly over the blemish. (Note: For best coverage, use a product with a thick consistency.) Smooth down gently and blend the edges. Apply regular foundation as usual.

When your complexion has too much red in it, use a green underbase toner (many cosmetic companies make them), and a beige foundation on top.

If your skin is too sallow, use an orchid shade underneath and pink or peach over it.

If your complexion is porous, uneven, or indented with scarring— other than acne pitting—use a cream blusher. It gives a smoother look than a powder one. Follow with powder blusher if you want to intensify

Going a Long Way on a Gleaming Smile

"Maintaining an attractive mouth is part of looking good after 40," says my dentist Cyndi Kulick, D.M.D., New York's Federal Plaza Dental Associates. "Tooth decay has all but disappeared by the time you're middle-aged, but it's time to check that fillings, crowns, and bridges are intact. And since some women develop a drier mouth after menopause, a condition that can cause tartar buildup, I would suggest that they have cleanings twice a year."

After mid-life you should consider increasing your calcium intake, says Dr. Kulick. "The same loss of calcium that can cause osteoporosis can cause a thinning of the bone that anchors your teeth." Don't let yellowish stains on your teeth detract from your face. Keep them clean. See your dentist regularly.

Teeth also need daily flossing and gums a daily massage. Cosmetic dentistry can usually correct chipped, crooked, or crowded tooth gaps; gold or silver fillings; misshapen or missing teeth; swollen gums; stained teeth; and very large or very small teeth. Dentistry can do much more these days than correct an overbite. If orthodontic work or cosmetic dentistry will help your teeth look better, consider it.

All this for the sake of a smile? Absolutely. A gleaming smile is one of your best assets. And as Dale Carnegie promised—he wrote paragraphs on the power of the smile—it wins friends and influences people.

---

color. But if you put dry makeup directly over moist, it will look blotchy; so dust on translucent powder between these two steps.

When your skin is deeply pitted with acne scars, use a makeup shade that is slightly darker than your complexion. A lighter shade will emphasize the pits. And use a powder blusher because a liquid will only get into the crevices and make them look worse.

If your skin is flawed (large pores, acne scars, or severe wrinkling), avoid brown blushers. They look muddy on flawed skin. Stick with warmer, pinker shades.

With severe wrinkling and acne scars, use makeup with a matte finish to tone down the *facial lines* and *small blemishes* that reflect light. With wrinkling, avoid heavy makeup, which clogs the lines and makes them more obvious. *And with acne,* use water-based makeup to avoid aggravating the skin's oily condition.

If a matte finish gives your face too masklike a look (this can happen when heavy opaque corrective makeup is used underneath), an opalescent dusting powder may help your complexion look more transparent.

MAGICAL MAKEUP MAKEOVERS
Jeanne Conlon, 44

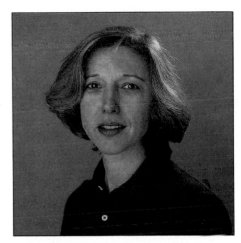

Jeanne played down her southern Italian looks and went for a preppy look. Makeup artist Peggy Esposito prescribed a trendier, more dramatic look, capitalizing on Jeanne's ethnic features, while minimizing the downward lines of her nose and eyebrows. Her deeply set eyes were shadowed and shaded upward to bring them out; the cheek area was made to look wider to minimize the broad jawline; the slightly broad nose was slimmed with shading applied just under the tip and down the sides. A mauve lipstick brought up the color of Jeanne's complexion. The sides of her hair were brushed up and held with a clip, the rest pushed back into a fastener, further de-emphasizing the nose and accenting the eyes. Add a single earring and a gray Italian silk shirt for drama. "I really *love* this look, but I hope my husband and son will approve. I'm not sure they'll recognize me."

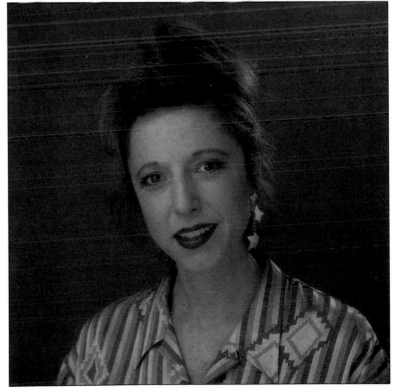

Sue Nirenberg, 50

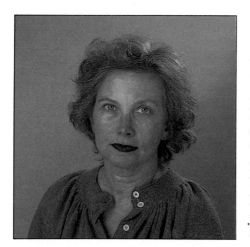

Sue's face needed color, and her lipstick was too dark. Her eyebrows were too heavy, adding to the downward lines of her face. Their color also aged Sue by contrasting too strongly with her face and hair. Her jowls also made her look older. Peggy Esposito applied a light pink base to Sue's face plus a pinkish coral blusher blended into her cheeks and the tip of her nose. A soft brown contour powder applied under the jawline maximized the jawline and minimized the jowls. The ends of the eyebrows were tweezed to create an upward line; black mascara made the upper lashes look thicker and longer. The lipstick was lightened to coral. The hair around Sue's face was layered to give height, volume, and lift to her face. Sue's reaction: "Once you know how much better you can look, it seems worth the extra effort to keep it up."

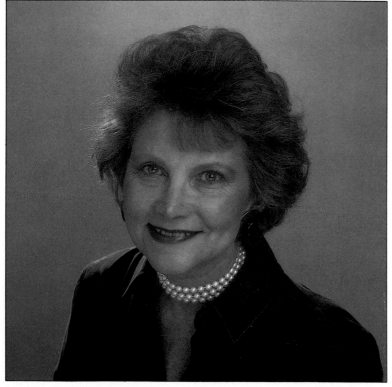

Abigail Thomas, 44

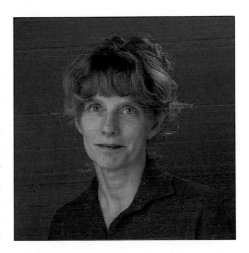

Abigail's prominent nose and good cheek-bones were being wasted, and her lovely skin looked too pale. Her thick, honey-colored hair needed "taming," said stylist Peggy Esposito. Concealer hid the dark circles under the eyes, and a peach-tone base plus translucent powder was applied to the face, then powdered peach blusher to the cheeks. Taupe-colored contour powder was brushed on under the cheekbones to emphasize their prominence. To make Abigail's nose appear narrower, taupe contour powder was applied to the sides and to the tip. Light brown eyeshadow was applied to the eyelids, and terra-cotta lipstick to the lips. The hair was cut in soft layers to shoulder length. "I wouldn't have believed my looks could change so much," said Abigail.

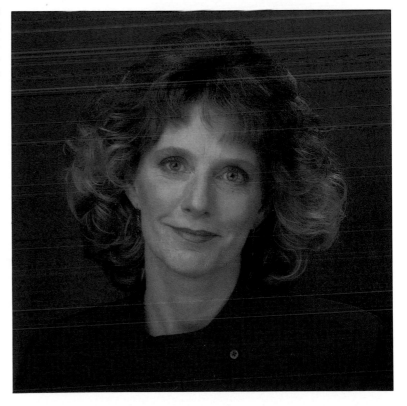

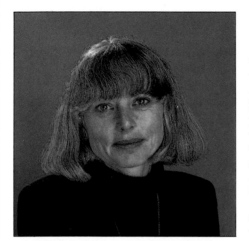

Elga Stulman, 53

Elga needed brighter makeup not only because of her olive complexion but because she wears a lot of black. Her long bangs concealed part of her eyes, said stylist Peggy Esposito. A pink-tone cream base was blended into Elga's forehead, cheeks, and chin, then translucent powder was brushed on. A mauve powder blusher was dusted onto her cheeks to brighten her complexion. The slightly broad nose was "slimmed" by brushing on a pink-tone contour down the sides. A light gray eye shadow applied upward at the corners made Elga's eyes stand out. A bright red lipstick gave her a brighter look. The bangs

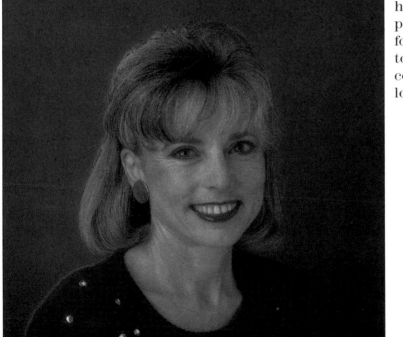

were lifted off her face to give her a more contemporary appearance. "I thought running four miles a day was enough to make me look healthy, but cosmetics have helped me to look even better," Elga said.

Liz Atwood, 46

Liz worried about laugh lines around her mouth, "whistle" lines over her lips, dark circles under her eyes, and looking too "bright" for her age. Makeup expert James Reda applied peach-tone cream concealer to minimize the dark circles, a peach-tone foundation, and finally a loose translucent powder. Next came a peach blusher for the cheeks. Liz's eyelashes were curled to make the eyes look more open, and a dark brown mascara was applied to thicken them. A soft look was given to the eyes with a blend of plum, taupe, and charcoal powdered eyeshadow applied to the lids. The new lipstick was coral. The hair set with hot rollers was brushed away from the face. "I think Jimmy has given me some pointers on how to achieve a more natural look," said Liz. "I like it."

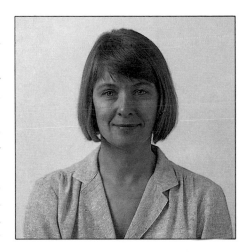

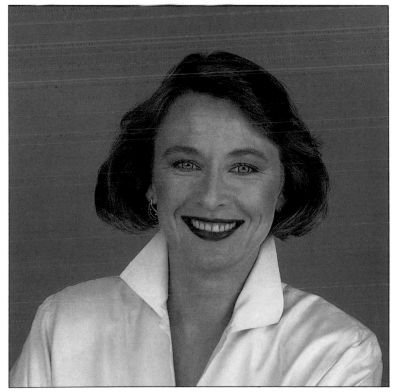

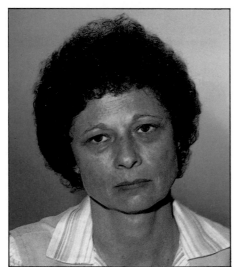

THE THERAPEUTIC POWER OF MAKEUP

Peggy Anderson, 45

People always asked me if I were tired, said Peggy, because I've had extremely dark circles under my eyes since I was a child. Linda Seidel, an expert in therapeutic makeup, used a coverup stick on those dark areas and blended it well. The important thing is to pick a coverstick to match your skin tone.

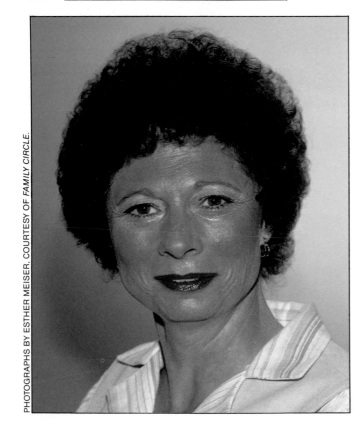

PHOTOGRAPHS BY ESTHER MEISER, COURTESY OF *FAMILY CIRCLE*.

Jane Badolato, 44

Jane came to Linda Seidel for therapeutic makeup on referral from a plastic surgeon. He felt that the injections needed to remove "spider veins" (broken blood vessels) in Jane's face would have left unsightly scars. The makeup worked. "I left with such a glowing complexion that I got compliments on the street," said Jane.

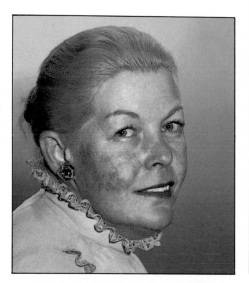

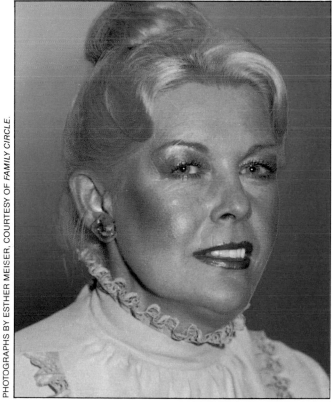

PHOTOGRAPHS BY ESTHER MEISER, COURTESY OF *FAMILY CIRCLE.*

Marilyn, 47: 20 Pounds Lighter and Feeling 30 Years Younger

If you can't imagine life without your old unhealthy habits—caffeine, junk food, alcohol, cigarettes (name your poison)—listen to New York actress Marilyn Rockafellow who is 47 and great looking. At 126 slim, trim pounds Marilyn weighs 20 pounds less and looks ten years younger than she did when I met her seven years ago. She was 39 when she started her diet and exercise program, which includes dancing, and quit smoking while doing it.

I found that it takes 30 days to break a habit, 30 days to develop a new me, and 30 more days to solidify it, so, when I wanted to quit smoking, I knew it would be a 90-day ordeal before I could even begin to think of myself as a nonsmoker. I didn't so much put pressure on myself to quit as psych myself into what I wanted, which was to quit smoking and not gain weight; in fact, to lose weight

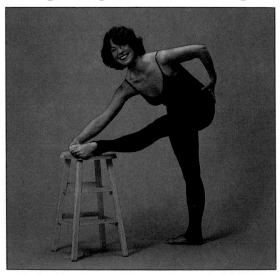

and feel good. Rather than concentrate on breaking the cigarette habit, I started a new habit, which turned out to be more enjoyable than the old one—and that was exercise. The only time I could exercise was early, before 7:30 A.M.

I finally decided that the only way I could really keep the momentum going was to use the buddy system. So I formed a pact with a friend. We agreed that we would meet at the gym every morning, and neither of us could *start* until the other got there. That way we each had a commitment to each other to make this new resolution work. Neither of us wanted to be responsible for the other's not being able to exercise, so I was spurred on by guilt.

My journal also reinforced me; I wrote something good in it every day about the way I was feeling. Instead of concentrating on how hard it was to give up smoking, I was praising all the enormous improvements in my health.

In an amazingly short time my body felt so much better, and I started to crave the exercise. This led me to want healthy food so that I'd continue to feel good. I started eating fruit, vegetables, pastas, grains, chicken, and fish and eliminated refined sugar and starches, meat, and oil. I also ate my last meal before 6:00 P.M. because I'd heard that it was harder to burn calories later in the evening.

I've kept up my new habits of exercise and correct eating, and I haven't gone back to smoking. Now I feel more energetic than I did at 16!

BLENDING

Use liquid foundation that blends easily and doesn't streak. Apply makeup with fingertips for a smooth, even finish.

Use soft, fluffy professional makeup brushes to apply powder. The smooth, natural look you can get with the right type of brush will make a big difference.

Blend color properly, especially to cover flaws well. Mix lighter and darker shades of foundation together in the palm of your hand; then pick up a dab at a time and gently smooth onto the skin.

Blend edges of your makeup carefully. This is especially important when your skin is blemished, as unblended edges of blusher could look like another scar or birthmark. Use a cotton ball to smooth large areas and a cotton swab for smaller ones like those around the eyes.

Match your face makeup to your neck color as closely as possible. When there is a difference between the two, bring the foundation down about 1½ inches on your neck, thinning it out little by little with a cotton ball as you move toward the edge.

CONTOUR

When one side of your face is fuller than the other, it can be made to appear slimmer if you shade it with contour powder, bringing color from under your cheekbone down toward the jawline. Look in the mirror carefully when you do this. The technique is tricky, however, and really depends on the contour of your face.

Keep the concept of light and dark in mind when contouring. Dark detracts light and will make an area appear to recede, while light reflects light and therefore will make an area stand out more.

To help mask a double chin, brush a little brown blusher from under your jawline down toward the center of your neck.

EYES

To widen close-set eyes, apply a light neutral shade of eye shadow to the inner corner of each eye, near the nose. Blend well. Put a dark neutral shade of shadow in the same area if eyes are too far apart.

If one eye is larger than the other, outline the upper and lower lids with eye shadow or pencil, making sure to draw a slightly thicker line around the smaller one. But never use a black liner; it's too harsh.

When you have dark shadows under your eyes, use powder eye shadow applied with an eyeliner brush as your undereye liner. A liquid or pencil would run and add to the problem.

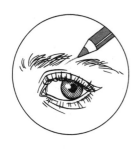

If you have scars on your eyebrows, use a sharp eyebrow pencil to fill them in. Try to duplicate the hairs in your brow by drawing short, feathery strokes in the direction of hair growth. Then brush over them with a powder brow makeup that you apply with a brush.

For eyes that are sensitive and tear easily, use nonallergenic makeup. Avoid mascaras with lash-building fibers in them. Don't use eyeliner inside your lower lids. And be sure to change your mascara tube every three months so bacteria doesn't have a chance to build up.

Look at fashion magazines for new ideas on eye makeup. Beautifully made-up eyes are one of the best distractions from a facial blemish.

LIPS

To a degree, the shape of your mouth can be built up or narrowed with a lip pencil. First, apply foundation to your lips as a base. Then use a shade of lip pencil that's deeper than your lip color. For a larger lip line, outline lips just outside the natural shape; for a smaller lip line, draw just inside the natural line. Fill in with lipstick.

TWO MIRACLE MAKEOVERS FOR SPECIAL PROBLEMS

Linda Seidel is a makeup artist who specializes in minimizing serious scars and birthmarks with makeup. But you can use her special tips when dealing with ordinary flaws. The therapeutic makeup she used in the following makeovers (excerpted from *Family Circle*) is called Covermark. (Note: Peggy Esposito also used it for the four makeovers on pages 135-38.) Covermark was invented 30 years ago by Lydia O'Leary who formulated the unique makeup to cover a flaw of her own—a port-wine stain, the name given to bluish red birthmarks.

Thick layers of regular foundation or theatrical makeup will cover flaws at first, but eventually a blemish will show through. Covermark, on the other hand, is waterproof. It will last through a humid day and several laps in a pool. Also you have a choice of ten shades that can be blended for a close match of your own skin color. Some makeup artists use other long-lasting makeups, such as Pan-Stik and Pan-Cake by Max Factor, to cover blemishes. And several makeup artists who have made a specialty of concealing serious skin flaws formulate their own cover-up products. At the time these makeovers were done, Linda was working on her own line. She is now marketing it.

Linda used this corrective makeup to make each individual's skin look as clear and natural as possible. Then she added the glamour touches because "beautifully made up eyes and lovely cheekbones and lips can do a lot to focus attention away from a facial flaw."

So expert has Linda become at the application of therapeutic makeup that she has given demonstrations before a board of plastic surgeons at Johns Hopkins Hospital. Many have sent her clients, feeling she does such a good job correcting problems. "No one is a lost cause, so don't dwell on your problems," Linda says. "Find a way to conceal them and go on to make yourself look terrific."

PEGGY ANDERSON, 45 (photos, page 140)
Extremely dark undereye circles:

First, smooth a vitamin E stick (available at natural foods stores) over the area. It will help the undereye cover-up stick, which goes on next, adhere to the skin better. Gently smooth the cover-up stick over dark areas, then blend well with fingertips. Make sure the color of the undereye makeup is close to your skin tone. Many companies make cover-up sticks, so experiment until you find the one that works best for you.

JANE BADOLATO, 44 (photos, page 141)
Broken blood vessels and blemishes where coloration is not distinctly different from the rest of the skin:

Use Covermark on flawed area only. Pat on over the blemish and blend the edges well with fingertips. Follow with a regular loose translucent powder to set. Smooth regular foundation over this and the rest of your complexion. Then apply blusher, eye makeup, and lipstick.

Disguising Serious Blemishes

To cover birthmarks, scars, and pigmentation problems, use fingertips to smooth Covermark over the entire blemished area, then blend edges well. Premix as many colors as needed in the palm of your hand until you get the right shade. To cover uneven pigmentation, you may need to apply a lighter shade to some areas and a darker one to others. If disfigurement is particularly dark or extensive, use the white finishing powder (also from Covermark) to set makeup and keep the scar or birthmark from showing through. Apply with a cotton ball; blot excess with a damp paper towel. Cover the unflawed part of the complexion with a mixture of Covermark and regular water- or oil-based liquid foundation—one that is light but gives good coverage. Sometimes regular foundation alone is better for the rest of the skin, so experiment. Last, apply blusher and eye makeup, blending to make skin look smooth and natural.

How to Choose the Right Eyeglasses

Eyeglasses! When I was a teenager, most of my friends and I would rather squint than wear glasses. Since those days, however, modern eyewear technology has come up with eyeglasses that can improve your vision and accent your skin tones and makeup as well.

Unfortunately, those of us who grew up with Dorothy Parker's painful axiom, "Men seldom make passes at girls who wear glasses," still don't think of glasses as an accessory. So we stay with a certain frame that sits comfortably on our noses and around our ears, and we change our lens prescription from time to time. We don't even realize that the frame may be outmoded and heavy. But a flattering frame can be had. Just follow a few rules that depend upon the shape of your face and the color of your hair and complexion.

Basic Facial Shapes and Frames to Flatter Them

There are basically four facial shapes—oval, round, square, and triangular (or heart-

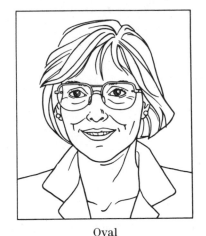

Oval

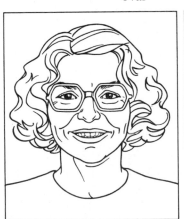

Round

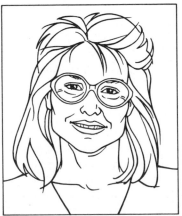

Square

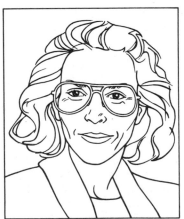

Triangular

shaped). If the shape of your face is oval (the cheekbones dominate), you can wear almost any kind of frame, including rimless and semirimless. If your face is oval but slender, choose frames that are heavier to fill out and balance the face. If your face is round (the greatest width is at the cheeks), it usually has no angles. Choose a frame that will give your face a slightly more angular look, but avoid any frames with harsh, exaggerated angles. Also avoid round frames that accent the fullness of your face. (A slightly wider frame creates a slimming effect.) If your face is square (characterized by a squared, angular jawline), choose a softer, more rounded frame to diminish the angularity of your face. To cut the width of the jawline and make your face appear more oval, be sure the outside corners of the frame extend out over your cheekbones. Gentle, easy lines with an upward sweep are flattering. If your face is triangular or heart-shaped (characterized by a very wide forehead and a narrow chin), choose a frame that is heavier on the bottom, as this brings some of the weight down toward the lower half of your face.

When you select frames, check them out for size as well as shape. How can you tell when the frame is too large or too small? *The frame is too large* if too much of the frame extends beyond your eyes on the side, if too much flesh shows under your eyes, if you can see your eyebrows through the lens, if the bridge of the frame doesn't fit securely on your nose, or if your glasses slide off when you bend your head forward. *The frame is too small* if the outside edges of the frame fall somewhere within the eye area, if your eyes aren't centered in the frame, if your eyes are cut off by the frame, if your eyebrows extend above the frame, or if your eyes overpower your glasses.

Choosing the Best Color and Shape of Frames and Lenses

The color of the frame is important, too. In general, as you grow older, you should stay away from bright blues, ruby reds, teal greens, black, dark tortoiseshells, yellows, golds, silvers, and metallic bronzes. But whatever your frame choice, there are tinted lenses that have excellent cosmetic value. Rose- and peach-tinted lenses camouflage puffs and bags and jowls. (Avoid light gray and green tints, which look drab and bring out lines and yellow tones in your complexion.) As we grow older and the angles of our face soften, the most flattering glasses—for everyone—are the new faceted tinted lenses that are lightly enclosed in metal clips and temples. Or you can select pretty pastel frames that convey the faceted shape with matching tinted lenses.

Even the temples (the frame sides) can flatter or detract from your look. Top temples tend to add a "lift" to your entire face and are especially good if your skin sags or droops. Fairly wide center temples attract attention away from the thickness of a lens.

(continued)

How to Choose the Right Eyeglasses—*Continued*

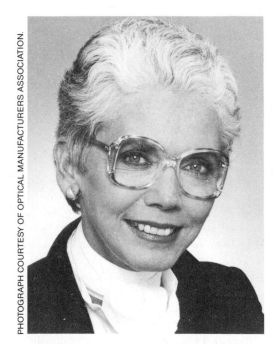

PHOTOGRAPH COURTESY OF OPTICAL MANUFACTURERS ASSOCIATION.

Note the gorgeous fashion eyeglasses with an outward sweep at the bottom of the lens to balance the angles and make the face look better proportioned. With a wide forehead and narrow chin, eyeglasses that stay within the temple hairline should be chosen. A light-colored bridge gives width to the eyes.

Wide bottom temples help to camouflage crow's-feet and lines that appear at the sides of the eye area. Stay away from temples with flowing lines in either plastic or metal or in combination.

When selecting glasses, remember that the top edges of the frames should form one clean line with the eyebrows. Avoid metal frame designs with colored enamel inlays, etched designs, or jeweled or hand-painted trims. (You're far better off concentrating on striking earrings than fussy frames to enhance your features.)

Makeup behind the Glasses

And don't think your makeup goes unnoticed behind your glasses. Skillfully applied eye makeup is more important than ever. Eye shadow and cheek color carefully placed can bring out the depth and sparkle of your eyes. So here are some general hints for making your eyes appear larger and more luminous behind glasses. To make the eyes seem farther apart, sweep the eye color up and out from the center to the outer corners of the eyelids. To make the eyes appear deeper set, apply the color in the eyelid crease area. In general, if you wear eyeglasses, apply your eye makeup a little more heavily than before you wore glasses. Makeup artist Gigi Williams says, "When you wear eyeglasses, you apply blusher the same way as when you're not wearing glasses—on the cheekbones. Blusher shouldn't go any closer to your nose than an imaginary spot in line with the outside of your iris and no higher on the cheek than the glass frames." If only Dorothy Parker could have known all this!

BEAUTY EXPERT IS QUIZZED ON COMMON MAKEUP MISTAKES AND WHAT TO DO ABOUT THEM

Jean Adams is a beauty expert and consultant who does makeovers all over the country and was *Redbook*'s beauty editor for 14 years.

Q. What are the worst makeup mistakes women over 40 make?
A. A lot of women let their eyebrows grow very thick so the brow overpowers the eye. On the other hand, some women pluck their eyebrows, so they're too thin, calling attention to themselves and not their eyes.

Q. Why is that so awful?
A. The eye itself, not the brows, should be the focal point. The arch of the brow should be over the iris of your eye.

Q. Tell me more.
A. Women tend to make pencil strokes too long and unnatural looking.

Q. What would look natural?
A. You shouldn't make one hard pencil stroke so that it looks like a nasty gash. Instead, you should feather in the pencil in short strokes so it looks natural. It's also a good idea for a woman to lighten her brows if they are much darker than her hair. It's a pain to keep up, of course, but it has a definite brightening effect, especially if her hair is bright.

Q. What about eyeglass frames?
A. Eyeglass frames should complement the eyebrow shape. Eyebrows should be under the top rim—not above or below it because that shortens the look of your upper face. If you have a small face, for example, don't overpower it with huge frames.

Q. What about the shape and color of the frames?
A. Most women choose frames that are too large and too harsh. They're not aware of light peaches and white frames, which are more flattering.

Q. More flattering than what, for example?
A. Tortoiseshell, which is hard for a lot of women. Black and brown tortoiseshell is often too harsh. You have to take hair color into consideration. Sometimes a woman will have worn black frames when she was younger, but then she'll color her hair and forget to change the frames. She isn't thinking about the balance of her total look.

Q. How does one choose the most flattering eye shadow?
A. So many women over forty wear eye shadow to match eye color, thinking that they're intensifying their eye color. Actually it competes with their eye color. A complementary shade plays up their own eye color instead of competing with it.

Q. For instance?
A. For instance, for blue eyes a lavender is flattering. Light pink intensifies blue eyes. Brown eyes with flecks of gold and green look browner and more glittering if you use a gold and green color. The eye shadow, you see, really creates a background for eye color.

Q. Can you explain further?
A. Most women think of eye shadow as color instead of shadow. What shadow does is call interest to the color and shape of her eye. A lighter color—say, a light pink or mushroom—helps the eye shadow adhere and evens out the skin tone of the lids, which get slightly discolored as we age.

Q. I've never managed to use eyeliner very well. I can't be the only one.
A. No, most women who learned about eyeliner in the sixties are still putting it on like a separate line, and it looks like a black slash. It's ugly, and it doesn't open the eyes as many assume—but closes them up. Instead of thinking of eyeliner as a line, a woman should apply eyeliner with a dot-dash (broken-line) deep into her lashes technique. Then she can connect the dots a little if she likes. Eyeliner was meant to intensify the eyelashes by becoming part of the base—not a separate line.

Q. Is there a trick to avoiding clumpy mascara?
A. To avoid clumping lashes, apply the mascara separately to each lash. This also works well if you have thin, skimpy eyelashes. Instead of using the eyeliner wand horizontally, turn it vertically, working at its tip. It takes a few more seconds, but it's worth it.

Q. Let's go on to the rest of the face. What are the mistakes you've seen there?
A. I've seen lots of red, red cheeks. Women wear too much rouge or blusher and it's distracting. The idea of blusher is to use it as color where you would blush naturally—on the tip of the nose and the cheekbones. It's a mistake to call too much attention to the blusher itself. And it's also wrong not to wear enough. The blusher must create a balance between the eyes and the lips.

Q. How should you select a blusher?
A. Blusher colors have to relate to your skin color and to your other makeup colors. If it's startling, it looks unnatural. Too much of a contrast.

Q. Do you see a lot of foundation mistakes?
A. Do I! Many older women apply so much foundation that it looks like a mask. Others don't match the foundation to the skin color. As a woman gets older, she doesn't realize her skin color has changed. She loses her rosy glow. Women should think of foundation as something that evens out skin color rather than as a cover.

Q. Do you think the more expensive makeup lines are better?
A. Some people may disagree with me, but I think it's worth spending money on a good foundation. There's definitely a difference in the blending of the ingredients for the foundation. You can expect to spend anywhere between $8 and $18 for a foundation. A good one will spread well over your skin. A foundation has to be the lightest possible texture. Discolored skin requires thicker applications—but not much. You should apply foundation with your fingers. Take a little out of the bottle and apply the dots where you see problems first and then even that out. Start in the chin area, then nose, then forehead, then eyes. Then look at your cheeks. Think of a foundation as a veil, not a heavy screen. You can mix foundation with a drop of water or moisturizer, but good foundations usually have a nice consistency.

Q. What about lipstick?
A. Some women over 40 are afraid of lip color because they learned about makeup in the sixties when lipstick was out of fashion. They don't wear enough to blend in with other makeup. Again, there has to be a balance with other makeup. On the other hand, too much lipstick overwhelms the rest of the face. As we age, the lip lines are less well-defined, so we use a lip pencil or lip brush to outline them and keep the lip color within.

Q. Any other mistakes over 40?
A. I see women at 11:00 in the morning who look as if they wore no makeup—it looks awful. Unkempt and ungroomed. It turns out they do wear makeup but it fades.

Q. How do you keep makeup from fading?
A. You have to reapply it during the day. It can't be helped. After you apply it in the morning, several hours later re-dab foundation on your

face, a little moisturizer on the dry places and beneath the eyes to spark them up. Reapply blusher. Lips get dry so you need to reapply protector and lipstick. The more carefully you apply the first time, the longer the lipstick will stay.

Makeup fades more quickly on older skin because it is drier, and dry skin absorbs makeup more quickly. Fading also depends on how much you touch your face. Constant touching—resting your face on your hands, for instance—takes makeup off. You can minimize fading if you use a good moisturizer and then powder over your makeup.

Do you remember my cousin, plain Martha, who yearned to look like Lana Turner? Well, Martha of the inky eyes and the stained brown legs has turned into a stunning woman in her late fifties. Her hair is the kind of gray that women envy, her once-scarlet lips are a lovely coral, and her cheeks are no longer bright with rouge but just touched ever so subtly with blusher. A corporate attorney who still runs two miles every day after work, Martha has finally come into her own.

UPDATING YOUR IMAGE

Chapter 6

The other day I was leafing through a pile of old photos, and there I was—this barely recognizable being—a wide-eyed, ingenuous, and definitely colorless young woman of 26. No character. No guts. No well-earned wrinkles. *Definitely no clothes sense.*

Not that I don't wish for the small waistline I had then. I do. But, over all, I think I look a whole lot better today than I did 22 years ago. If I were to meet now the person I was then, I'm sure I would be bored to tears with her.

If you'll allow yourself to admit it, I think you'll find that you, too, are more interesting looking than you were 10, 20, even 30 years ago. Or at least you might be if you gave yourself a chance.

Unfortunately, at our age most of us encase ourselves in the image of our youth—the preppie (then it was the Peck & Peck) look of '65, '59, '53, or '48. Or we settle into what *McCall's* fashion editor Zazél Loven calls the cast-iron, pale blue polyester pantsuit. This middle-age uniform is still one of the hottest-selling items on the market today; certainly its popularity is not due to the chic image it projects. It sells because of the lack of imagination that leads us to buy it. This tendency we have to dress "in our youth" or dress too sensibly and unimaginatively makes us look older than need be.

What we need to do is put together an adult look that projects the image of the women we are today. At last, we can look like the women we've always wanted to be (no, not Elizabeth Taylor; no, not Linda Evans). I mean it's time to explore the woman we've harbored inside all these years and never really let out for countless reasons—our efforts to fulfill someone else's expectations of us, or maybe a fear of our own sexuality.

Of course, bringing out the woman inside isn't easy, particularly if you've kept her hidden for years. Dr. Mara Gleckel, a New York psychotherapist, specializes in helping women find this inner person through a series of exercises we'll present in these pages. I attended Mara's workshop with six other women, and the first exercise given was one called Nickname. We were asked to give the name we thought best expressed our inner selves.

Helen, 49, the mother of adult children and newly married for the second time, called herself "lively." Helen was, in fact, matronly, even dowdy—certainly not lively looking. The view she conveyed to the group definitely collided with the way she saw herself.

After a little probing, Helen admitted that she had a great deal at stake in making her current marriage work. She was hesitant, she said, to make herself look too attractive (*and* too sexy) because she felt it would conflict with her concept of being "a good wife."

Elga Stulman, 53: A Style of Her Own

Over the years, since age 20, my hair has become gray. During those years, I didn't know what to call my hair color. Now that I *am* gray (and by the way, I like my gray hair), I no longer wear the muddy colors I used to wear—the beiges, browns, and taupes. Now I stick to three colors: black, gray, and red.

Just recently I've become aware of what does look right on me, and I like my wardrobe better than ever. I've developed my own sense of style. I no longer believe in the myths about small women—that small women shouldn't wear shoulder pads, or big bags, or big jewelry, or big skirts, or long jackets.

Four or five years ago, my look was undifferentiated because I stuck by the rules. Recently I've become braver. It helps to have a 17-year-old daughter to inspire you. She bought one of those 1950s fake leopard-skin coats—remember, the ones we thought we'd never wear again.

Well, I bought an updated version from Europe on sale for $200. I wear it with a red hat. Hats—they make everything look terrific!

Clearly she had quite a way to go to make anyone think she was lively, much less too sexy. Dr. Gleckel advised Helen (Lively) to make changes gradually. "You don't have to do it overnight," Helen was told. "You can be a loving, supportive wife at the same time you're emerging with more vibrance, and your husband won't feel threatened."

Shortly after our workshop, Helen had her dowdy (but naturally curly) mop revved up to a wilder and livelier hairstyle, which was converted to a vivid auburn with henna.

What was the outcome? A few weeks later, Helen reported to Dr. Gleckel that her husband *loved* her new look. He liked the idea that other men found Helen attractive! He had taken her out for dinner and dancing and had teased her about the approving looks she received.

The exercises we did during the workshop helped bring each of us closer to the woman we wanted to be, while shedding the image of the one we had felt we were *supposed* to be.

The next exercise was this: Imagine you have entered a forest and suddenly come upon a stone wall. You want to get to the other side. "What do you do?" The responses were as varied as the women in the group. One wanted to know more about the wall: "How high is it?" "Is there a way to go around it?" "What is it made of?" She was thinking of looking for handholds as a way of climbing up the wall. Failing that, she thought she might try to find a rope, throw it over the branch of a tree, swing to the top of the wall, and then slide down the other side. Another woman said she would first make sure there was no way around the wall, then she would check carefully to see if there were any openings farther along where she might pass through. My own reaction was simple. I'd get over the wall, no matter what. It was there so I had to get over it. It never occurred to me that I didn't have to. Clearly there were several ways of dealing with this wall—including mine.

The way each of us approached the wall, of course, shed a little light on our inner selves, an aspect that had a lot to do with the image we projected to the world. Clearly I could be identified as a rock, as in "solid as a . . . ." And I wasn't so sure, in my heart of hearts, that I liked the image—L.L. Bean backpacker, I'd call it. What I sent out were messages of independence, of not really needing any help. And I wonder why no one comes to help me.

The next exercise we did showed us how we often let ourselves get stuck in the past through school, marriage, and parenthood. If we were a tomboy, rebel, good girl, or bookworm to our parents, we may have carried that identity into the present, even though we might be quite eager to shed that image today. One woman, who wanted to be Lily, but looked like Rock, said that good girl was probably her childhood image. The leap from good girl to rock seems like a natural course of events. Both childhood and adult images had pushed Lily out of the way.

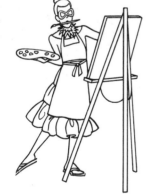

I too had been good girl as a child . . . and had graduated to being a rock. The person I really wanted to be was artsy craftsy, the kind of woman who paints, makes pottery, goes barefoot (lives in the country, of course) and cooks big, hearty soups. The fact that this fantasy bears slight relationship to the life I actually lead now is unimportant. What is important is the knowledge that there is a part of me that would like to be artsy craftsy. So there should be a part of her in the image I project.

Are you catching on? Have you figured out what you would do should you come to a stone wall? Have you given a nickname to who you were as a child? Have you thought about the name you would choose to express the woman you would like to be today?

YOUR COAT OF ARMS

Here is another exercise that will open you up to a better understanding of who you are now, where you are in terms of goals and accomplishments, and where you want to be. Draw a shield like the one on opposite page. Divide it into six parts. And fill in each section using pictures or key words.

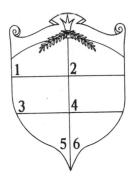

✔ In section 1, show your greatest achievement to date, in any area—school, home, job, love, etc.

✔ In section 2, indicate your greatest failure.

✔ In section 3, show two things you would like people to remember about you.

✔ In section 4, draw a picture symbolizing a part of your life that is important to you, one that most people don't know about.

✔ In section 5, draw a picture of your most important goal.

✔ In section 6, draw a picture or think of a word that summarizes what you would do if you had only one year left to live.

It's amazing what a few minutes with a little diagram can reveal about you.

This last exercise helps put into perspective the importance of getting your goals and your image into alignment *now*. Take a piece of paper and draw a line across it. On the left-hand side, write your birthdate. On the right-hand side, write the year that ends your normal life expectancy. Then put a dot on the line indicating where you are now in that span of years.

1946 ————————————●———————————— 2026
(40 years old)

Then ask yourself: How much time have I already lived? How much of it was spent doing what was expected of me? How much time do I have left to get my M.B.A., own a plant shop, adopt a child, go to Tibet, write a biography, redecorate my house, buy a farmhouse, put together the fabulous wardrobe I've always wanted? It puts things into perspective, doesn't it?

Hopefully the exercises designed by Dr. Gleckel have helped you gain some insight into who you *really* are, so you can update your image to reflect the real you. Perhaps her questions that follow will help you even more.

SELF-ASSESSMENT EXERCISE

This exercise (which you should do alone) will help you step out of yourself and take a good look at how others see you. It will help make you aware not only of what you see but whether you like what you see.

In this exercise we are concerned with individual characteristics that make you unique. In everyday life, much of our self-evaluation is based on external roles or categories we fall into. We say we are mothers, wives, lawyers, teachers. But telling someone that you are a secretary, a mother of two, and divorced doesn't go very far toward describing who you really are. It doesn't tell someone whether you're sympathetic and kind or withdrawn and cold; whether you're enthusiastic or shy; ambitious or lazy.

When Americans meet in a social situation, "What do you do?" is almost always the first question asked. It defines a starting point for a conversation and sometimes helps people quickly find out if they have any common interests. But it also points out that we live in a culture where inner realities are often ignored. So it is even more important that we take time to sit down and take stock of ourselves. Because whether or not we choose to talk openly about our inner selves, we consciously or unconsciously send out messages about who we really are every time we move or open our mouths or put on a different blouse.

This exercise is divided into parts. The first part has to do with how you see yourself. The second with how you think others see you.

A. WHAT ARE YOUR ASSETS?

1. I think I am
   (a) attractive   (b) unattractive   (c) passable

2. My clothes are
   (a) chic   (b) dowdy   (c) average

3. In my work I am
   (a) creative   (b) unimaginative   (c) one of the crowd

4. Intellectually, I am
   (a) smart   (b) dumb   (c) average

5. As a conversationalist, I am
   (a) exciting   (b) boring   (c) able to hold my own

6. The way I live my life is
   (a) adventurous   (b) cautious   (c) sensible

7. When I talk, I am
   (a) listened to   (b) ignored   (c) tolerated

8. At a party I am
   (a) eager to meet new people   (b) hesitant   (c) very uncomfortable

B. WHAT DO OTHERS THINK OF YOU?

1. In your present or most recent relationship, is the man someone
   (a) you chose   (b) you felt you should choose   (c) you had no other choice

2. Do your sexual relationships
   (a) last   (b) have a short life   (c) don't occur

3. Do you have the job
   (a) you want   (b) settled for what you could get   (c) can't get a job

4. If you have a problem
   (a) are there one or more women you can confide in   (b) don't share your problems   (c) have no one to talk to

5. In a crowded department store, are you
   (a) waited on quickly   (b) waited on by turn   (c) the last one waited on

6. Are you
   (a) frequently complimented on your looks   (b) often mentioned in terms of your looks   (c) constantly hear others get all the praise

7. In a group do people
   (a) turn to listen to you   (b) interrupt   (c) go on speaking as if you hadn't spoken

8. Do people
   (a) confide in you   (b) rarely ask for your opinion   (c) turn to someone else for advice

Scoring:

For part A: If you have six to eight (a) answers, you have a very positive self-image; if you have six to eight (b) answers, you have a negative self-image and don't find yourself very interesting; if you have six to eight (c) answers, you have a rather colorless self-image and have settled for being mediocre.

For part B: If you have six to eight (a) answers, the response of others shows they think you are as terrific as you think you are; if you have six to eight (b) answers, people aren't paying much attention to you; if you have six to eight (c) answers, your low self-image causes others to respond to you negatively.

Your scores on part A and part B should be within a few points of each other if your self-image matches the impression others have of you. If the scores are not approximately the same, you are not successfully communicating your image of yourself to others. Go back and pinpoint those areas where the greatest differences occur. For example, if you are attractive, smart, and creative, why can't you get a job or manage to get waited on in a department store? If your scores are much lower in part B than they are in Part A, you are hiding the best parts of yourself. Your rewards in life will be greater when you can communicate your positive qualities to others. On the other hand if your scores are much lower in part A than in part B, your low self-image is not in line with reality. Others recognize your good qualities. Accept the fact that the image you project is you.[1]

CHOOSING YOUR FUTURE ROLES

By the time a woman reaches mid-life, she has played many roles, gathered many images of herself. It is her privilege, at a certain point, to decide which roles she will continue to play and which she will shed.

At mid-life, you are freer both physically and mentally to be the woman you want to be. Your children are usually old enough to care for themselves unless you are one of the many women (many of them my friends) who have opted for late motherhood. Either way, the point is that, hopefully, you are now doing what you *want* to do with your life.

One way to gain a sense of how you use your time is to draw a circle, then cut it into wedges indicating the proportion of time that you spend doing different things in your current routine. Make a wedge for time spent on housekeeping, on career, on relaxing with family or friends, on whatever occupies you on a daily basis. For comparison, make another "pie" showing how your time was occupied ten years ago. Now make a third "pie," subdividing it into sections that indicate how you would *like* to be spending your time now or in the near future. Does that give you a

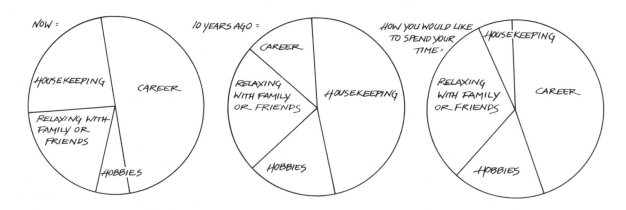

1. The information on self-assessment exercises on pages 157-59 is reprinted from *Ego, Image and Success* by Mara Gleckel and Muriel Goldfarb (Brooklyn: Long Island University Press), reprinted by permission of Mara Gleckel.

Try to Get a Concept of Yourself

Whenever Barbara Walters, ABC-TV journalist, feels a need to rev up her self-confidence, she repeats to herself: "I am the way I am; I look the way I look; I am my age."

Aside from having a personal motto to cheer her on, Barbara Walters presents herself with such assurance because she takes the trouble to make herself attractive. In her book, *How to Talk to Practically Anybody About Practically Anything* (New York: Doubleday & Company, 1983), she states her belief that "the way you dress is the billboard that tells perceptive people how you feel about yourself." But women often concentrate on what they feel are relatively unimportant details, like matching up accessories or getting the right hem length, instead of making an effort to express a point of view or create a personal image in the way they dress. Of course, be conscious of your silhouette, but don't waste energy trying to compensate for a figure or facial defect that can't be changed. "Try to get *a concept of yourself*," she urges. "You're an individual and not someone stamped out of a mold in a doll factory."

clearer sense of how you use, or should use, your time to best advantage? Think how you might rearrange the "pie" wedges to organize a life that will be more fulfilling to you.

Remember the lifeline you were asked to consider earlier? Well, consider it again!

HOW TO FIND THE RIGHT IMAGE FOR YOU

"Sixty percent of what people take in is your body language, 30 percent facial expression and a key part of that is your hair, makeup, and the way you dress," says Dr. Gleckel. "Only 10 percent is what you say or sound like."

Psychologist Judith Waters, who teaches at New Jersey's Fairleigh Dickinson University, goes along with this: "Society has determined that certain looks have certain meanings," she says. "It may not be fair, but it's reality." So, give your best image the go ahead!

There is no rule of thumb about how you should look except your own. You know—or at least have a glimmer of who you are on the inside. What you want to do is get your outside appearance to fit more closely with that inner person. Dr. Gleckel has some definite ideas on how to go about it.

1. First, think over your relationship with your mother. Are you acting out her fantasies or your own? Are you using your life to act out the goals she missed in hers? And in doing so, are you suppressing your own desires? Are you hiding your real self?

2. Analyze why you have your particular look. Do you, for example, shun makeup, or the color red, because your mother told you it was frivolous? Do you wear a certain hairstyle or clothing style because you looked that way when you met your husband? You may discover that your reasons are faulty—and that's the first step toward changing.

3. "Look at your own fantasies and find the fine red line that runs through them," says Dr. Gleckel. "In your daydreams are you soft and feminine, when in real life you're tailored and conservative? Imagine the way you'd like to look, then start concentrating on clothing, hairstyles, and makeup that reflect that look."

4. Pay attention to the messages you get from others. Do people treat you as if you weren't too smart? Do you hear, "Don't worry your pretty little head," when you want to seriously discuss the problem at hand? Are people who don't know you well surprised when they learn certain things about you? Write down these reactions from others and study them; then decide what you need to change to get the reactions you want.

5. Determine your major goals, then your minor ones, and apply this information to your image. For instance, if you want a new or better job, perhaps you should try for a more businesslike, self-assured look. On the other hand, if you want to expand your circle of friends, maybe you should have a warmer, more approachable look.

6. Verbalize your present image, but state it in the past tense. "When you say, 'I was too cutesy or wishy-washy or bland,'" explains Dr. Gleckel, "you're already on the way to getting rid of that image. Then state your preferred image in the present tense—'I am vivacious, competent, and poised.' This helps you to see yourself differently."

7. Think about the outfits you feel best in. What is there about them that makes you feel good? Next visualize the outfits you have and ask the same question. The answers will give you a clue to your best image.

8. In addition, you might want to pick a woman you know, or someone on television or in a magazine, who looks the way you would like to look. Analyze how she achieves her look, pick it apart, look at all the elements—the shoes, the jewelry; whether she wears a hat. Then try to instill these ideas into your image.

9. Go to department stores and try out different looks. Go to different departments within your old familiar store. Don't get stuck in a rut. Experiment. Don't reach automatically for the nice, neat, little silk shirtwaist dress. Try on the royal blue beaded dress. Try on new accessories—a variety of them. When you go shopping, wear an outfit that will be a backdrop for the accessories, so you can see how they really look.

This "shopping" expedition will be just for browsing—to get ideas, to see what might suit the image you want to project. Now go home and see if parts of that image aren't hanging in your own closet, undiscovered.

THE CLOSET CATHARSIS

It's amazing how many changes in my life have been initiated by my cleaning my closet: getting rid of a man in my life who was doing me no good, starting with a new and better one; getting out of a job that was doing me no good, starting with a new and better one.

There is no better way to begin working on your new image than to ransack your closet. Rethink all the clothes that don't relate to the emerging new image you've set for yourself. Be firm with yourself. Let these four rules guide you:

1. If it doesn't fit, get rid of it. You want a wardrobe for the size 10, 12, 14, or 16 you are now, not the size 6 or 8 you might once have been and, face it, may never be again.

2. If you haven't worn it for two years or more, find another home for it. It probably is out of style, was never right in the first place, or doesn't suit the image you want to project today.

3. If it doesn't go with anything you own or are likely to purchase, you don't need it. You want things that mix and match in a variety of ways. That will be your ultimate goal in building your new wardrobe. You want it to fit together in a jigsaw puzzle (well almost). Always leave room for almosts.

4. If it bothers you because it's too itchy, too weird, too worn out, or whatever, eliminate it. If a garment merely needs altering, mending, or cleaning, put it aside. But get it fixed. Don't let unwearable clothes mess up your new image and clutter up your life.

Stephanie Winston, an expert on organization and the author of the book *Getting Organized* (New York: W. W. Norton & Company, 1978), cautions against pulling everything out of your closet at once. A better approach, she maintains, is to take things out one by one, evaluating each item in terms of what it does for you and how much you need it for the type of life you lead. (A woman who spends winter weekends in the country doesn't toss out a perfectly good down parka because it's not the right color—this is one of those almosts in your jigsaw puzzle.) Ms. Winston suggests having two boxes at hand, one marked Give Away, and the other Throw Away. You might consider getting together with a friend of the same size, who is interested in streamlining her image, too. Your "giveaways" could become her new look. Or, like my friend Harriet, organize a clothing swap among several friends of different sizes and types. And I, personally, would call the Salvation Army or other charitable organization before I'd throw anything away. You'll get a tax deduction, which is a bonus.

Put together different combinations of the clothes you decide to keep. Then you might want to arrange them into four categories as Stephanie Winston does.

1. For the top half of the body (sweaters, light jackets, blazers, blouses, shirts)

2. For the bottom half of the body (slacks, skirts)

3. For the whole body (dresses, suits)

4. Special occasion wear (your ballgown, perchance)

A BARE-BONES WARDROBE

Out of the clothes you decide to keep—after your closet rampage—single out those that will work best as backdrops for accessories. There is no quicker way to arrive at a new look than through the right earrings, scarf, belt, hat, handbag, or bracelet.

Now let me introduce you to Lawson's Law of Elementary Fashion. I base this on the assumption that, unless you are wealthy enough to own several designer dresses, it is more practical to have a wardrobe made up of separates. Three of each—blouses (or shirts), sweaters, and skirts make at least 9 outfits. Interchange pants with skirts if you like, or add three pairs of pants to make at least 12 outfits possible.

Select these separates in three colors—one your primary backdrop, say, for your pants or skirt; the other your secondary color, say for a shirt; and the third color an accent to appear in a scarf or as the color of your jacket.

I like to wear black, but a black dress with a lipstick-red jacket. My third color is gray (or silver) and sometimes white. So I'll wear silver

---

Avoid the Color Clothing Box

Sherri Austen is an image consultant and color analyst who gives workshops in the New York area. She points out a mistake we frequently make in buying clothes. "Middle-aged women like to wear colors they feel safe in," says Sherri. Time and again they choose beige or black because they regard those colors as neutral. "Instead of building a stunning outfit based on a choice of pants in a flattering color, like wine or marine blue, they buy black pants, thinking they'll go with everything." Sherri refers to this as getting into a clothing box and advises women to take a close look at themselves, to study their figures and coloring, and then build a wardrobe based on those "givens," not merely the "safe" colors.

What Clothes Tell Us

The clothes you wear, of course, tell people a lot about you. In the book *The Language of Clothes* (New York: Random House, 1981), author Alison Lurie tells it like this:

"Long before I am near enough to talk to you on the street, in a meeting or at a party, you announce your sex, age, and class to me through what you are wearing—and very possibly give me important information (or misinformation) as to your occupation, origin, personality, opinions, tastes, sexual desires, and current mood .... By the time we meet and converse we have already spoken to each other in an older and more universal tongue."

loop drop earrings (remember I want to look a little artsy craftsy) and sometimes a long white scarf.

You need not confine yourself to the obvious background colors—black, brown, burgundy, and navy. You might choose variations like camel, rust, or marine blue. I know an attractive gray-haired artist who uses royal blue as both her basic and background color. She wears it with black with an occasional touch of white. I also have a friend who uses turquoise as a basic color or an accent for everything she wears. She even has turquoise boots in the softest Italian leather. Another friend has picked dusty rose. If it's not in the color of the blouse she is wearing, you'll find it in her belt, her scarf, or her shoes. Dusty rose is as much a part of this friend in my mind as her signature, which is very loopy and rather rosy, too.

As I've been saying all along, it is terribly important to express your inner self in the things you wear—to give clues about the person deep inside you. With some practice you'll be able to do this while projecting a totally integrated look. Part of the secret is remembering that "less is more." Nothing belongs in your wardrobe that does not work with several other things you wear, and nothing belongs there that doesn't say something about the *real* you. Now it's time to go shopping, but before you do, think about the following.

COLOR MAKES ALL THE DIFFERENCE

"The right choice of color in clothing and makeup can make you look younger, prettier, thinner, more successful, and save you money," says Jennifer Morris, a color and style consultant who heads It's Your

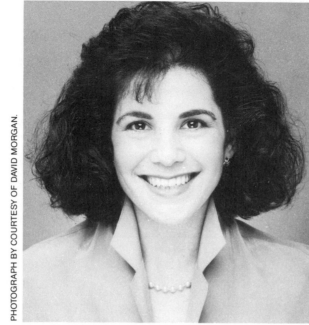

PHOTOGRAPH BY COURTESY OF DAVID MORGAN.

Jennifer Morris

Image on New York City's Madison Avenue. Jennifer studied with, and is certified by, Fashion Academy, Costa Mesa, California, which is the alma mater of Carole Jackson, author of *Color Me Beautiful* (New York: Ballantine Books, 1981).

Jennifer tells me that the basis of the season (Winter, Summer, Spring, and Autumn) color theory that is currently so popular was pioneered by Gerrie Pinckney, one of the founders of Fashion Academy. The seasonal color concept was actually mentioned over 50 years ago, when Johannes Itten, a European artist, noted that some students chose colors in harmonizing groups that generally fell into four categories. He labeled the color groups with seasonal names. Ten years after Itten's discovery, Marjorie Bliss Nebeker and Suzanne Caygill, both from San Francisco but working independently, divided the personal color of clients into four groups, two warm and two cool, and continued using the seasonal names. The colors from Winter and Summer form the cool group, while the warm colors are found in Spring and Autumn. Nebeker and Caygill were concerned primarily with cosmetic application. Pinckney extended the concept into a total wardrobe plan.

According to the noted American colorist Albert Munsell, there are five basic primary colors: red, yellow, green, blue, and purple. Everyone can wear these five colors, depending on the undertone, value, and clarity. The undertone is determined by the amount of blue or yellow in the color (blue-gray as opposed to dove gray); the value is the lightness or darkness of the color (powder blue versus navy blue); and the clarity is whether the color is clear or muted (clear pink or dusty rose, for instance).

Your most becoming colors are determined by the color of your skin, eyes, and hair. "You should wear your colors, rather than your colors 'wearing you'," says Jennifer.

WINTERS

Wardrobe colors for Winters are true or have a blue undertone and are vivid and clear. They range from very dark, like navy or royal purple, to very light, icy tones. Winter women wear the strong, bold colors, as well as black and chalk white; shades of gray from charcoal to very pale; gray-beige (taupe); lemon yellow, from bright to light; emerald and pine green, from bright to light; true green, from bright to light; aqua to hot turquoise, Chinese blue, royal blue (can be very purple), true blue and navy—all from bright to light; royal purple (violet), hot pink, magenta, cerise, azalea, fuchsia, bright burgundy, blue red, and true red—all in shades from bright to light.

Accessory Colors for Winters

Black, navy, gray, maroon, white, and gray-beige are all accessory colors for winters. Accessory colors can also be any bright or light color within the Winter palette. Shoes should be the same color or value as your hemline, or darker. Your bag should be the same color or value as your shoes, or lighter. Shoes and bag need not match, but must harmonize. Hose should be light to dark gray-taupe or rose-beige, sheer gray, navy or black, or the icy tones. These shades should each harmonize with shoes and hemline.

Makeup Colors for Winters

Included in the makeup colors for Winters are foundations in rose tones of beige or tan; cheek colors of wine, rose, or red; and lipstick and nail colors in true red, blue reds, or pinks.

SUMMERS

Summers' wardrobe colors have a blue undertone and are soft pastels to dusty, dark shades. When colors are medium to light, they can be dusty or clear. When medium to dark, they should be dusty. Colors include shades of mauve or rose-brown; shades of blue-gray—light through medium charcoal; dusty blue, grayed blue (cadet), sky blue, medium blue, powder blue, grayed navy, periwinkle blue, and aqua; pastel to deep blue-green; eggshell white; shades of banana yellow; shades of lavender, orchid, plum, grape, wine, raspberry, burgundy, cordovan, maroon, rose-pink, and medium to deep pastel pinks.

Accessory Colors for Summers

Navy, wine, gray, rose-brown, rose-beige, and gray are the accessory colors for Summers. Summers should follow the same advice given to

---

How to Find the Right Colors for You

Put a check by the skin tone, eye color, and hair color that best describes you in each season. If none of the choices is correct for your coloring, leave the section blank. The season in which you've been able to check all three categories—your skin tone, eye color, and hair color—will most likely be yours. You will need a good light and a close friend to help you be objective.[1]

WINTER

Winter Skin Tones	*Winter Eyes*	*Winter Hair*
__ White	__ Light to dark brown	__ Platinum blonde
__ Light to deep rose-beige	__ Black-brown	__ Golden blonde
__ Brown	__ Olive brown	__ Golden brown
__ Brown-black	__ Olive green	__ Medium to dark brown
__ Black	__ Gray-blue	__ Chestnut brown
	__ Gray-green	__ Brown-black
	__ Turquoise	__ Black
	__ Dark blue-violet	
	__ Hazel (combination blue, green, brown)	

SUMMER

Summer Skin Tones	*Summer Eyes*	*Summer Hair*
__ Fair with pink tone	__ Clear blue or gray-blue	__ Light ash blonde
__ Light to medium rose-beige	__ Clear green or gray-green	__ Medium ash blonde
__ Deep rose-beige	__ Aquamarine	__ Light to medium ash brown
	__ Hazel (blue-green with brown or yellow flecks)	
	__ Soft, cool brown	

---

1. Reprinted with permission of Fashion Academy, Costa Mesa, California.

Winters for matching shoes with hemlines and matching or harmonizing bag with shoes. Hose should be light tones of taupe, rose-beige, sheer gray, navy, or the icy tones. They should harmonize with hemline and shoes.

Makeup Colors for Summers

The makeup colors for Summers include foundation shades in natural, pink- or rose-tone beige; cheek colors in pink, rose, or wine; and lipstick and nail colors in pink and rose, mauve and plum, burgundy and wines.

SPRING

Spring Skin Tones	*Spring Eyes*	*Spring Hair*
__ Pale ivory (may have rosy glow)	__ Light to dark blue	__ Flaxen blonde
__ Golden ivory	__ Blue-gray	__ Golden blonde
__ Pink or peach (may have rosy glow)	__ Green-blue (aqua)	__ Strawberry blonde
__ Deep peach	__ Gold-green	__ Light to dark golden brown
__ Light to medium beige	__ Light gold-brown	
	__ Topaz-yellow	
	__ Hazel (combination blue, green, brown)	

AUTUMN

Autumn Skin Tones	*Autumn Eyes*	*Autumn Hair*
__ Ivory	__ Light to dark brown	__ Honey blonde
__ Light, medium, or deep peach	__ Red-brown	__ Strawberry blonde
__ Light, medium, or dark beige	__ Olive brown	__ Bright red to deep auburn
__ Reddish	__ Golden green	__ Light to dark brown with gold or red highlights
	__ Hazel (brown with blue-green)	__ Deep chestnut brown
	__ Turquoise	

SPRINGS

Colors that are most becoming to Springs have a yellow (warm) undertone. They are warm, clear, medium to light, fruity or flowery colors: dove gray, light to medium; milk-chocolate to beige shades; bronze to clear camel; shades of buttercup yellow, light gold, maize, and cream; shades of apricot, tangerine, salmon, peach, and coral; poppy red; medium violet, periwinkle blue, and royal navy to sky blue; shades of aqua from clear and light to warm and bright; shades of clear yellow-green, lime, and celery green.

Accessory Colors for Springs

These accessory colors for Springs are navy, milk-chocolate, camel, warm gray, and yellow-bone. The same rules for shoes and bags apply as for Winters and Summers. Hose should be nude shades, ivory, light beige, light suntan, sheer navy, and the icy tones of warm colors. Hose should harmonize with shoes and hemline.

Makeup Colors for Springs

Springs should select foundations of ivory, beige, and peach tones; cheek colors in peach, coral, or clear red; and lipstick and nail polish in peach, coral, toffee, watermelon, or poppy red.

AUTUMNS

Wardrobe colors for Autumns are yellow, muted earth tones: warm browns, beiges, and oyster whites; camel and butterscotch colors in shades from light to dark; rusts; chrome and taxi-cab yellow, canary yellow, golden yellow, and daffodil; all shades of orange, pumpkin, apricot, terra-cotta; orange-red, tomato red, and bittersweet; corals, dark to light; shades of warm green including olive, jade, pea green, and khaki from dark to light; teal, turquoise, and periwinkle blue, from dark to light.

Accessory Colors for Autumns

Dark brown, rust, camel, medium brown, olive, and off-white (yellow-bone) are the accessory colors for Autumns. Shoes should be the same color or value as hemline, or darker. Bags should be the same color or value as shoes, or lighter. Hose may be nude, warm beige, golden suntan, sheer brown, or cinnamon. Light pastels to match or harmonize with hemline or shoes should be in warm tones.

Makeup Colors for Autumns

Included in the makeup colors for Autumns are foundations of ivory or peach tones in beige or tan; cheek colors in peach, coral, or amber; and lipstick and nail polish in tones of golden orange, orange-red, orange-rust, or brick red.

Because both Winters and Summers are cool seasons, silver accessories are more complementary to their skin tones. Gold is better on the warm seasons (Springs and Autumns).

Colors that may be worn successfully by all seasons include eggshell, coral, aqua, and periwinkle blue.

The ability to see color is an art. To be certain of your season, you may benefit from the help of a certified color consultant. Use the accompanying chart as a guide in determining your season. Remember, whatever your season, you are not limited to just a few colors. There are over 10 million colors, which gives you at least 2½ million to choose from!

40 WAYS TO SAVE SHOPPING MONEY WHILE YOU WORK ON YOUR IMAGE

Today, a trip through any department store is a shock. Skimpy dresses go for mucho dinero. A winter coat takes a week's pay (sometimes two weeks'). Outfitting teenagers is an inhuman task. Is there a way to beat it, we wondered? Then we investigated and found there are countless ways to hold down rising clothing costs. And they start with you. Because the first step is to get hold of your own look.

1. Budget how much you can spend.
Have some idea of what you *can* afford before you enter a store. It will help your self-control.

2. Make a list of what's needed.
Keep it in your head or in your wallet. This will help you avoid impulse buying and give you direction when you walk into the clutches of a department store. It also helps you not to pass up a good buy when you see it.

3. Go through your closet.
Try on everything. See what fits and what is drastically out of style. Put different combinations of clothes together. Throw out garments you haven't worn over the past year—ones that are too itchy, too weird, or too worn out.

4. Shop at quiet times.
At the dinner hour and early in the day fewer people are in the stores. When you're less rushed and hassled, you're likely to make better decisions.

5. Plan ahead.
Hurrying out on a Saturday afternoon to buy a dress for that night is a mistake. If you do want to buy something new right now, make it a small item: jewelry or a belt. A garment bought in panic is regretted in leisure.

6. Read.
Check a few fashion magazines before shopping a sale, and you won't get stuck with last year's duds. *Consumer Reports* and its annual

What Three Fashion Experts Suggest to Update Your Wardrobe

"Buy a blazer, it will make everything else you have look new," says Carrie Donovan, fashion editor for the *New York Times*. She also thinks buying a pair of shoulder pads is a good idea. "The newest fashions have broader shoulders, so stick the pads into your sweaters, blouses, and dresses to change their silhouette."

If you want to build on the blazer, fashion consultant Irene Satz suggests adding a skirt that's not too full and a V-neck, ribbon-knit pullover to wear with it.

Emily Chou, New York City image consultant, recommends an inexpensive Indian caftan for evenings. "Decorate it with glittery braid and rhinestones," she says.

---

buying guide issue give advice on the durability, workmanship, care, and appearance of standard clothing brands. The International Fabricare Institute (Doric and Chicago Avenues, Joliet, IL 60434) offers 78 different "Facts About Fabrics" leaflets. Be as specific about the type of fabric as possible when you send for any of them. "Your Clothing Dollar" (available at a nominal fee) is a 40-page booklet full of savings ideas offered by the Money Management Institute (Household Finance Corporation, Department FC 2700, Sanders Road, Prospect Heights, IL 60070). Write for current price and shipping costs.

7. Get salespeople to know you.
Salespeople usually work on commission and are eager to help steady customers. Tell them your tastes and needs. Ask them to put aside a certain pair of shoes if they come in or let you know if a coat you like goes on sale. Telephone for standard items like your favorite underwire bra and have them charge and send it or mail it C.O.D. Remember, time is money.

8. Look for comfort.
No matter how wonderful the garment appears to be, if it makes you itch, or it binds, or you swelter in it, it's no bargain. When you try it on, consider how it really feels. Sit down in it, raise your arms, bend over in it in front of a mirror.

9. Shop off the beaten track.
Army & Navy stores sell wool 13-button sailor pants, pea coats, and army fatigue pants in 100% cotton. *The dime store* has great cotton bikini panties, white Fruit of the Loom T-shirts (great with shorts or to sleep in), and plastic summer shoes in red, green, blue, and other Lifesaver colors. *Riding shops* let their tweed hacking jackets go at half price twice a year. They last a lifetime and make great all-around sport jackets. Classic English-style riding boots are also a good buy, as are rain ponchos. *Ethnic shops* (East Indian, Moroccan, Polish, Chinese) sell caftans, peasant blouses, and kimonos, often at amazingly low prices. *Sporting goods stores* sell parkas at 50 percent off in the summer. And year-round their parkas are usually cheaper than those at department stores. And don't miss their webbed belts and sweatpants.

10. Try thrift shops, flea markets, garage sales, and church bazaars.

I buy my lingerie at New York's Park Avenue Church of Our Savior's annual church bazaar. One of their members is evidently a corporate mogul of a big lingerie company. A year's worth of brand-new bras and panties costs me only $30. At the same bazaar I also bought an Oscar de la Renta jacket for $3 and a very chic red dress, which took me through a holiday in St. Johns, the Virgin Islands, for the steep price of $1. (Okay, I bought $55 earrings to go with it.) At the Girl's Club of America Thrift Shop on 77th Street in Manhattan, I have bought hand-knit sweaters and Shetlands for as little as $3 and a Turnbull and Asher shirt (imported from England and very expensive if you buy them on Fifth Avenue) for $3. Reptile-skin belts go for $1 to $3. Designer eyeglasses, Yves St. Laurent, Anne Klein, and Gucci are $2 to $5. Put lenses ground to your own prescription into the frames. I once bought a beautiful pair of ankle-length boots (never worn) for $5 at a garage sale. The same boots had sold at a New York Madison Avenue bootery for $200.

11. Haunt the outlets.

Conditions here tend to be rough. You may have to try on clothes in a large open warehouse, in the midst of packed clothing racks and people. And they'll take only cash to avoid the service charge on credit cards. But the savings are worth it, as prices are rock bottom. Most book stores now sell shopping guides that give you the lowdown on local outlets—where to find them and what to expect. Each place is different, but generally they sell clothes that were overstocked or cancelled. *Factory outlets* sell directly from the manufacturer at near wholesale prices. *Wholesale outlets* are operated by middlemen who distribute clothes to the stores from the manufacturer. Savings are up to 50 percent. *Importer outlets* deal in French, Italian, Spanish, or English clothes selling at about half the retail price. Discount shops offer clothing bought from several manufacturers so you'll have variety, although goods may not be from the current season. Markdowns are 20 to 30 percent.

12. Buy from local craftspersons.

You get expert workmanship at a good price, especially if they work out of their home, with no middleman or shop rent to pay. Good bets are: leather hats, belts, crocheted caps, knitted sweaters, jewelry, and metal buckles. Look for these artisans at craft fairs and flea markets. Or write to your state arts council (c/o Crafts Coordinator) for a list of them.

13. Shop wholesale.

Occasionally manufacturers sell to the public, mostly on Saturdays and almost always for cash. Sometimes you may just happen to hear about it, but more often you will find out about such a source through a friend's recommendation.

14. Shop store closeouts.

Here you get the merchandise that didn't sell the first time around because it had a ripped seam, missing buttons, was slightly shopworn, or was an off color. The garments may be brought in from one or a number of stores owned by the same corporation or family and sold at one place. Hart Schaffner & Marx's big sale at their Chicago warehouse is a seasonal roundup of leftover merchandise nationwide from their retail stores. Or the clothes may be pulled from within the store itself and sold in a special place like Filene's famous basement in Boston.

15. Shop resale stores.

Usually these are designer clothes that belonged to socially prominent women and have been worn but once or twice. They sell at half price, and the original owners share in the receipts.

16. Build around one basic color to wear year-round with two accent colors.

Choose black, beige, brown, burgundy, gray, or marine blue. Pick two accent colors that enhance your own coloring. My basic color is black. I accent with red or gray. So I'll buy black pants, a gray sweater, and maybe grab a black and red scarf. Get the picture? This helps you structure your wardrobe so you don't go astray and overbuy.

17. Take high fashion in small doses.

If you have a craving for the new and outlandish, satisfy it with a small representative accessory. If it's 1987 you might indulge in a pair of beaded drop earrings or pull out a rhinestone pin from 1955 and put it on the lapel of your tweed jacket.

18. Buy classics.

They have a timeless appeal and don't become quickly dated. Simple basic styles are wardrobe expanders (straight or dirndl skirts, a basic long-sleeved cashmere or lamb's wool sweater, a tweed blazer, a knitted vest, one-color silk blouses, a basic black wool or cotton dress) because they can be dressed up or down, depending on the occasion, and readily coordinate with other garments. A black velvet blazer, for example, goes with a skirt, a silk dress, or a pair of tweed slacks.

19. Mix and match separates to extend your wardrobe.

For example, three each of blouses, pants, sweaters, and skirts, make 12 outfits.

20. Select garments to go with those you already have.

Never go for 100 percent change; that's expensive, unless money is not a consideration for you. Instead, integrate new garments into your present look piece by piece. Everything should fit together like a jigsaw puzzle. Anything that doesn't fit in was probably a mistake. It is wiser to give away that mistake than try to add to it, increasing your wardrobe to unwieldy proportions.

21. Set your own style.

Everyone is different in size and shape, not to mention personality, life-style, and interests. Clothes that "aren't you" are going to hang in your closet. And that's a waste of money. The smart shopper looks at the latest fashion trends and picks only those that are becoming to her, changing them with personal touches until they fit her own personal needs. Getting your own look takes a lot of fighting it out with the mirror. And ultimately, it means fewer clothes taking up space in your closet, but more that work.

22. Don't dress strictly by the season.

Build your wardrobe around a core of fabrics and styles that work as well in June as in January. For example, look for a black knit dirndl skirt, a red caftan sweater, a black polo shirt, a white cotton turtleneck, and khaki cotton pants. Such multi-season items are perfect for those odd but inevitable—unseasonably hot (or cold)—days in any climate.

23. Layer and unlayer.

If you buy all-season cottons, you can layer them with wool sweaters and shirts, trapping warm air between them for added warmth. They're actually warmer than a single, heavy, bulky item of winter gear. On a really cold day start with thermal underwear underneath everything and you can get by without a winter coat. Layer heavy knee-length socks and leg warmers; wear a pair of crepe-sole shoes if you can't afford winter boots. In summer, unpeel the layers. Put the khaki cotton pants with a number of colorful T-shirts and work through the hottest months; wear the black cotton skirt with a cotton summer knit top.

24. Stretch your wardrobe with accessories.

Put espadrilles with the khaki cotton pants in the spring, loafers in the fall. In April, add a crisp hanky to the pocket of a tweed blazer, and wrap a large muffler around it in October. Replace the paisley scarf you've worn all day with jewelry at night, and dress up a basic black dress.

(continued on page 179)

UPDATING YOUR IMAGE
Helen Poulas, 49

Helen said she thought of herself as "lively," but she certainly didn't look it; matronly, even dowdy, was the image she conveyed. Her concept of being a good wife conflicted with Helen's desire to appear attractive and sexy. She came closer to being the woman she wanted to be by dismissing her false ideal that equated good with plain. An exciting new hairstyle and a freer way of dressing were expressions of a new attitude that allowed Helen to show her true self-image.

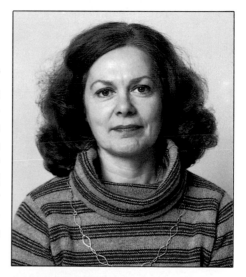

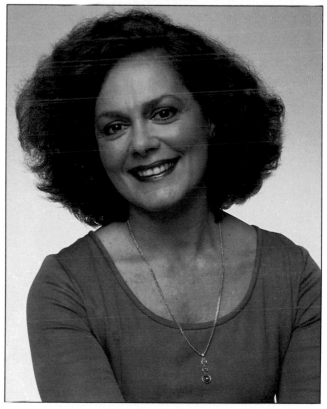

Molly's Makeover

Molly had plenty of clothes and good taste. Her clothes were made of quality fabrics, and they were all well cut. But in her heart she harbored a desire to look a bit more dramatic. She fantasized herself as the center of her own salon, where artists and literary people would gather in the manner of the late nineteenth century.

But no hint of the dramatic Molly showed on the outside. Her choice in clothing was conservative in color and style. We had to get Molly to "step out," so we sent the very imaginative Holly Shapiro, a fashion stylist, to invade Molly's closet. Both Molly and Holly were very brave.

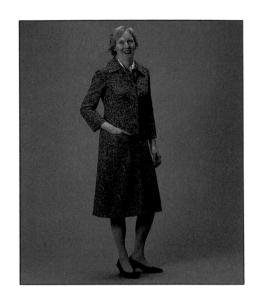

Together they hauled clothes out of Molly's closets and drawers. Then Molly began to try on the new combinations Holly worked out. She put together outfits that Molly had never dreamed of wearing—and they all came from what she already had in her closet.

"Molly was used to combining clothes and accessories with caution," said Holly. "She'd put together a cream-colored blouse with any color skirt, because it was safe. I showed her that you could take a forest green skirt, a turquoise blouse and an olive sweater, and put that all together with a pink scarf and it would work."

Molly would take no chances, Holly explained. She would wear a single necklace next to her neck under her open shirt, one bracelet, and a pin on the side of the shirt. Holly showed Molly that piling on the necklaces and bracelets would make a dramatic statement. She showed her how to button up her collar and wear the necklaces over the blouse and under her collar—and to pin her blouse together at the throat with a pin. The necklaces could be wrapped, as well, to give them more bulk.

Molly is 5 feet 10 inches tall, so she was afraid of all "that bulk" in jewelry and in clothes because she felt it made her look larger. In truth, Holly explained, larger, bulkier jewelry, bigger, bolder clothes, and dramatic statements like wearing a hat worked better with Molly's size than snugly fitted clothes and understated jewelry and accessories.

Layering was a concept Holly introduced into Molly's wardrobe. As you can see in Molly's "before" picture, she is wearing a simple tweed dress. In her "after" picture, with new makeup designed by Gigi Williams, she has explored new clothes and made a grander statement with layering. The clothes all came from Molly's closets and drawers with the exception of the shawl. This was actually a throw Holly pulled from the back of Molly's sofa.

"You have to begin to look at everything you have with fresh eyes, even your interior decoration," said Holly, who now had Molly trying on her husband's Stetson hats, his scarves and mufflers, his sweaters, vests, and shirts to great effect.

Molly's large tweedy tunic had been given to her, but she had avoided wearing it thinking it was too bulky. She had certainly never worn this tunic with a skirt—the skirt was usually worn with a particular sweater that was almost the same shade. The hat was worn only with her coat. But Holly felt she looked so sensational in the hat (in fact, any hat) that she could wear it with pants and look very stylish.

A muffler wrapped around her neck and fastened with a pin was not anything Molly would ever have worn either. But she saw, with Holly's guidance, that this too looked dramatic and worked wonderfully with her height. Of course, bracelets were piled on with this outfit—many of different colors bone, brown, and pink.

Molly's stockings in the photo are gray and worn with wine-colored shoes. "Women should have a wardrobe of stockings in different colors," said Holly. "Your stockings should never be darker than your shoes. It's also important that your stockings coordinate with your shoes first, and then the rest of your outfit." Don't, for example, wear blue stockings to match your blue dress if your shoes are wine-colored—better that the stockings be wine-colored, too.

Holly also cautions women to put as much care into what they wear on the "outside"—their coat, scarf, and hat if it's winter, their raincoat in the spring—as what they wear on

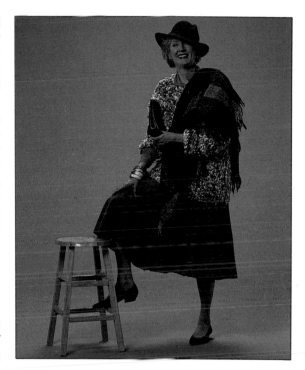

the "inside." Women will get all dressed up and then just throw something on top. They presume that no one will see them in that something. But there are all those people who see you coming and going. "Pay attention to your outerwear," Holly says. "Make sure the scarf looks good with the coat, and the hat looks good with eveything."

"Molly had a desire to be more exotic," says Holly. "There was fire going on under that quiet surface, and I wanted to bring it out in her clothes."

What Should Every Woman over 40 Have in Her Wardrobe?

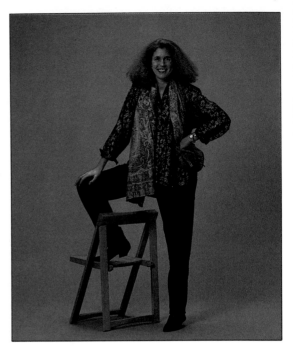

I asked Zazél Loven, *McCall's* fashion editor, for expert advice on assembling some basic wardrobe elements that will take you just about anywhere. Here are her valuable suggestions—just in time for your next shopping expedition:

✔ You need a good jacket that is not part of a suit. It should have a squarish shape and fall below the waist to the hip. In the winter I'd make that a tweed jacket; in the summer a linen blend. Get a black velvet jacket for evening wear.

✔ For outerwear, I don't think you can do much better than a basic chesterfield, straight-line coat.

✔ If you wear slacks, choose the kind that fall straight—no gimmicks—and wear them with low-heeled shoes. I'd get the slacks in a dark color.

✔ When it comes to a *great* wardrobe, less is more. After you've dressed, look in the mirror and see if you can't remove two things. Usually you can. Go for fewer but better clothes. *Fit* and *fabric* mean more as you get older. It's also better to dress in an understated way. For example, a black wool crepe dinner suit—in fact, any thing in black with an accent of color looks fashionable. Tweeds are nice as long as they aren't matched.

✔ To complete the perfect over-40 wardrobe, you'll want a gray or black pleated skirt to go with your three-quarter-length jacket, a charmeuse silk shirt in a white or creamy color (even a polyester charmeuse will do; some are quite nice today), a long sweater vest, a couple of big square scarves (dark paisley is always in style), and a good large leather shoulder bag.

✔ When you shop for these wardrobe basics, you don't have to spend a lot of money. You should get to know your local off-price stores (around here it's Marshall's, Loehmann's and T. J. Max). You should always add to your wardrobe in terms of what you already have. Don't end up with a closet full of clothes that don't go together.

25. Buy boots in sturdy leather, classic styling, and a neutral color.
Taupe, tan, and wine always look more expensive than black and blend with a variety of wardrobe colors. When you try on boots, be sure your toes are comfortable as feet swell when you wear them. Be sure that the heel doesn't slip up and down as you walk, causing blisters, and that the stitching will hold up. If the boots aren't lined, run your hand inside to check for rough seams.

26. Look for more than one use for each garment.
One shirt layered over another serves as a light jacket. A cotton knit dress worn over pants makes a tunic. A black V-neck T-shirt with a piece of jewelry at the neckline can be worn with pants or a skirt for an evening out. In the summer wear the same top with a printed cotton skirt, and it will take you anywhere. It also goes over jeans or a swimsuit, and you can exercise or even sleep in it. A long cotton T-shirt worn with sandals substitutes for a bathrobe and bedroom slippers.

27. Get a good leather bag.
Don't skimp on workmanship or price. Keep it simple: no fancy clasps or a lot of metal. Get good leather if you can afford it. The idea is to have a bag you can use for years. This is worthy of a major investment, but you can manage without breaking the bank. Early January is a good sale month for bags, at 50 percent off the original price.

28. If you can't afford leather.
Get a canvas bag. Keep it in a basic style and color; no darling felt flowers or stenciled mottoes. If it's leather trimmed, all the better. But vinyl is passable if it's simple and sturdily sewn. One of the best buys around is a Danish schoolboy's book bag with lots of compartments, which can be ordered for $18 plus $1.50 mailing cost from Chocolate Soup (249 East 77th Street, New York, NY 10021). Or get a woven African basket shoulder bag with leather handles, the kind Diane Keaton wore in *Annie Hall*.

29. Substitute a full-length yellow boating slicker for expensive rainwear.
You not only save on the initial cost but on cleaning and waterproofing bills later.

30. Limit the amount you spend on clothes you will wear infrequently or those that wear out fast.
This includes party clothes, dressy shoes, and play clothes.

31. Buy on sale.
With good planning you can purchase clothing at the end of one season and put it away for the next. Savings run as high as 50 percent. Store-wide clearances are held after Christmas and after July 4th. January is the best time to buy handbags; January-February, skiwear. If you get there early on the day of the sale, you have a wider selection of sizes and styles and colors. Budget your clothing wardrobe with these seasonal sales in mind. But, be careful about buying high-fashion colors and styles on sale; they may be dated the next season.

32. Buy clothes that fit properly.
Never get a size that's too small thinking that you'll lose weight. If you decide to buy a garment on sale that's too big, consider the price of alteration to see if you'll really save any money.

33. Check the workmanship of the garment.
Are there wide seams and hem allowances? Are the seams smooth? Is the stitching even and close together? Are buttonholes sewn through on both sides of the cloth? Are buttons, snaps, trims, and zippers properly placed and securely fastened?

34. Comparison shop.
If you don't have time, get an idea of how your local store marks up by reading ads and asking friends. Why help to cover the cost of the chandelier or the carpets on the floor by paying high

Calendar for Shopping Sales

JANUARY
Costume jewelry, dresses, furs, handbags, lingerie, shoes, sportswear

FEBRUARY
Hats, sportswear

MARCH
Hosiery

APRIL
Women's and children's coats, dresses, bathrobes, hats

MAY
Handbags, bathrobes, lingerie, sportswear

JUNE
Dresses, bathrobes

JULY
Swimwear (after the 4th), handbags, lingerie, hats, shoes, sportswear

AUGUST
Swimwear, furs, women's and children's coats

SEPTEMBER
Accessories

OCTOBER
Hosiery, bathrobes

NOVEMBER
Women's and children's coats, dresses, bathrobes, shoes

DECEMBER
Women's and children's coats, shoes

---

prices in a fancy store when a plainer store may sell the same clothes for much less? Learn the various departments within a store. See what type and price merchandise each carries. A similar outfit may be a much lower price in the sportswear department or the basement of the same store.

35. Buy standard clothing items at chain stores.
Because regional and national chains do an enormous business, manufacturers are eager to run off a special order of many thousands of units, producing T-shirts or terry-cloth bathrobes with the same technology that goes into clothes they make for more expensive retail stores. And you get a bargain: expert work and good fabrics at a low price.

36. Look into clothing seconds.
If the flaw you find can be easily disguised or mended, you may have a steal on a garment. Some stores, like those that sell skiwear or outdoor clothing, often have special Saturday sales on slightly damaged garments. The values are terrific.

37. Shop by catalog.
It saves you time and energy, both worth money to busy women. The prices also beat most. For example, right now, J.C. Penney Company is selling a tan leather pouch bag for $17.00, and L. L. Bean, a navy and white, heavyweight, water-repellent, 80 percent wool Norwegian fisherman's sweater for $28.50. Send to Freeport Maine 04033 for the L.L. Bean catalog. Ask for Penney's catalog at their local store.

38. Collect business cards.

Pick them up at boutiques, craft fairs, and flea markets, on your travels or while browsing locally. On the back of the card, write the prices and descriptions of the articles you like but want time to think about. Later, you can whip out your card and call or write the person who gave it to you. This foresight saves time and legwork.

39. Consider the value-per-wear of the garment, not only the price.

If the dress costs $150, it may still be a bargain because you know you'll wear it constantly. A $50 dress you settle on may turn out to be a one- or two-shot deal because you won't be as happy wearing it. Consider your satisfaction value into the cost.

40. Lose weight and exercise.

Thin women look better in clothes, whatever the price. And they fit into small sizes that go on sale at big reductions because fewer people fit into them.

PERSONAL SHOPPERS

If you are thinking about making additions to your wardrobe, a personal shopper can spare you the anxiety that often goes along with a shopping expedition. You can probably find one through or at your favorite department store.

You know the feeling that comes from spending hours flipping through clothing racks to find only two or three items you like. Then, there's going inside the dressing room for a face-to-face or rear-end-to-rear-end view of yourself in the mirror. By this time you look more haggard than usual. You may be made painfully aware that your legs are too short, your upper arms too flabby.

In your determination to find *something* that looks nice on you, you may have difficulty remembering what you were looking for in the first place. This won't happen if you put yourself in the competent hands of a personal shopper. You can tell her at the outset what you need and how much you are willing to pay. After a little discussion to determine how you live, your tastes, and how you want to look, the P.S. (Personal Shopper) will make a handpicked selection of items that will neither embarrass nor exhaust you in trying them on. And you may even love them. I did when I discovered my personal shopper in New York City's Lord & Taylor.

Shopping with a personal shopper is almost magical. So soothing to your nerves and at many places—at least at the ones where I've shopped—the service is free. You may also learn a great deal that is useful in the clothes choices she makes for you and the reasons for the choices. Through my first personal shopper experience, I learned that both Calvin Klein pants and shoes were a terrific fit for me—the best I ever found.

Whether you are shopping alone or with an expert, make sure you are feeling rested for the occasion. You are more likely to make a sound decision about whether to buy or reject. Remember, wear underwear, stockings, and the right shoes for trying on the clothes you need to buy. Trying on a dinner dress with a pair of sneakers is not an inspiring experience.

FAMILIAR FASHION FAUX PAS

Before you go shopping, make a mental list of the mistakes women our age tend to make:

✔ **Wearing Synthetic Fibers**

Unless they are blended with natural fibers, they tend to look cheap. (And sometimes even blends can look cheap.) Clothes made from synthetics seem mass-produced; you know that 5 million other women across America are wearing the same thing you are. And they cling. The convenience of being able to toss them in the washing machine means little if they don't look good on you. Also know that synthetics trap body heat, don't breathe, and are especially uncomfortable for women going through menopause with hot flashes.

✔ **Wearing Clingy Clothes**

Avoid pants, dresses, and sweaters that show every figure flaw. A tight fit is really a fashion "don't" for women over 40. Instead, choose roomy shapes and fabrics made to move with your body, not hug it. I think the naturals—silks, cotton, linen, or top-quality wools—as well as rayon are your best bets. I know a woman in her fifties who has an ample figure, with a capital A. But she also looks terrific in her glamorous and ample tunics, which she wears with nicely tailored slacks and her handsome silver Navajo bracelets.

✔ **Wearing Body-Baring Clothes**

Stay away from clothes that bare too much upper arm, midriff, chest, and thighs—unless you are blessed with upper arms, breasts, a middle, and thighs that are as tight and toned as

a drum in a naval corps band. Of course wear a bathing suit (one piece, unless you're Jane Fonda) and shorts. You're not a nun. But skip the miniskirts.

✔ **Wearing Clothes That Accentuate the Waistline**

Those of us who don't work out as often as Jane Fonda and Shirley MacLaine probably don't have the same waistline we had in the 1950s when we wore cinch belts and poodle skirts. Wear clothes that glide along your waistline, not grab it. Vests, cardigan jackets, and loose sweaters look good on most women over 40. On the other hand, overblouses can look as dowdy as white cotton gloves. Don't wear white cotton gloves, either. If the kids want to do it for what they call "retro-fashion," let them. They are imitating the fifties fashion; you should be escaping from it.

✔ **Wearing the Wrong Size**

You're not expected to wear the same size you wore at 25. Buy what fits you now—in the waistline, shoulders, around the hips, in the bust. Don't wear your clothes *too* short, even if you have gorgeous legs. Anything too short or too small tends to make women look older, not younger.

✔ **Being too Trendy**

Nothing is worse than trying to look trendy after the trend has passed. Show that you're "with it" by choosing an up-to-date

Camouflage for Over-40 Figure Flaws

Let's face it, over 40 everything seems to get bigger: waist, bosom, hips, thighs. This is not always true if you exercise regularly and eat right. But if you've let yourself go and you need to disguise a few problems while you get back into shape, here's what to do:

✔ Make sure your clothes fit. If you are a size 16, wear a 16; don't pour yourself into a 12. Trying to wear a smaller size only makes you look bigger.

✔ Avoid front-pleated trousers or dirndl skirts that add pounds.

✔ Avoid bold patterns. Plain colors are better.

✔ Don't wear clinging fabrics or too tight sleeves. Don't bare your upper arms; wear long sleeves in summer and roll them up.

✔ Add softness and color at the neckline to draw the attention upward away from your "weightier areas."

✔ If your waistline is thick, definitely don't wear belts. Don't wear a color that breaks at the waist—a pink blouse, say, with a gray skirt.

✔ Wear a long jacket, tunic, or vest to hide a thickened waist. Here you *can* wear a belt because only part of it will show through in the front.

✔ If your stomach sticks out too much, avoid fabrics that cling. Instead, wear A-line skirts—and skirts or trousers with diagonal-slash side pockets. A-line skirts also diminish wide hips.

✔ Long jackets, vests, and tunics will also hide heavy hips. Wear your skirt long enough to balance out your hips.

✔ Wear narrow belts, never wide ones that will emphasize your hip width. If your shoulders are narrow and your hips large, wear shoulder pads to even out proportion.

✔ Cover a large behind by wearing tunics over pants.

✔ Wear crisp fabrics—linens, wool serges, and gabardines. If you are overweight and out-of-shape, soft fabrics—jersey, chiffons, tissue woolens—will make you look puffier.

✔ Pastels, except when worn in limited areas, will also make you look heavier—sort of like a large ice cream sundae.

accessory—a leopard spotted scarf, or an art deco belt. If you want to buy something trendy like a leopard fake fur, don't spend your life's savings on it because you may want to chuck it the next season.

✔ **Not Paying Attention to Details**

Pleats and tucks in the right places can flatter you. (Always check them out in a three-way mirror before you buy.) In the wrong places, they accentuate your weaknesses. Ruffles, too, no matter how tempting can draw attention to a less than streamlined figure.

✔ **Wearing "Outfits"**

Remember your mother saying, "Think in terms of the whole outfit." Well, forget she said that. That meant, a dress or suit with matching handbag, shoes, and gloves, maybe a hat and appropriate jewelry, which was usually pearls—pearl earrings and pearl necklace. It was a package, a set that was trotted out "as is" for church, job interviews, and lectures. It was a perfect replica of the way the store outfitted the window mannequin. There was no room to maneuver, to add a different colored handbag or hat that might hint at who you were. Now think of French women who have a few carefully selected "staples," which they accessorize so skillfully they are suitable for any occasion. Nothing says middle-aged more than an outfit that is as obviously planned. Those "little dresses" that come with their own jackets spring readily to mind. Avoid them. They're good for first ladies or Margaret Thatcher to wear.

A FASHION EDITOR DISCUSSES COMMON WARDROBE MISTAKES

Zazél Loven, 40, *McCall's* fashion editor, talks about the mistakes she has seen along the way and tells what you can do to avoid them.

Q. What are the worst mistakes women over 40 make?
A. Right up front I can name two dreadful mistakes women over 40 make: (1) *dressing too young*—trying to look like the female superstar of the decade—in the 1980s that would be somebody like Madonna—and (2) *not keeping up with your grooming*—not doing your nails or having your hair cut when it needs it, not keeping your clothes pressed, your shoes heeled, your makeup fresh. (Have a makeup lesson if you have never learned how to apply it properly.)

Q. Any other mistakes?
A. Yes. Wearing too-short skirts or any top that reveals your midriff bulge! Fluffy knits like angora! Wearing anything that is too decorated!

Q. Is that all?
A. No. Another serious mistake is what I call "getting caught in the fast-freeze of the forties or fifties." You know, Peter Pan collars, pedal pushers, headbands, pageboys, or anything that looks cute and perky—vintage Doris Day or June Allyson.

Q. I have a feeling you have more mistakes on your list....
A. Yes. Overblouses! And the powder-blue, "bulletproof," polyester pantsuit worn by an astounding number of middle-aged women across the country. It looks middle-aged...it shouts middle-aged. It should be retired. Actually I'd skip all pastels, especially in the winter, unless I lived in the South or in a really warm climate.

Q. And?

A. Well, busy prints! Garish colors! Overly decorated handbags—the ones with seashells on them. And bulky tweed suits that make you look like Margaret Rutherford on a Miss Marple toot.

Q. Any basic mistakes in dealing with figure flaws?

A. Women rely too much on their imagination in deciding what an outfit does (or does not do) for them. First and always, look in a mirror (ideally a three-way mirror) at home or when you shop, to see how things look on you, and what the line looks like when you put different garments together. Be careful of your underwear. You want it to give your clothes a smooth line. You don't want it to show through. You don't want to see bra lines and panty lines under your clothes. A bra-slip is probably a good idea because it gives a smooth line. Legs look better in sheer stockings and a slight heel. Three-quarter-length vests do a lot to camouflage a thick waist. But, as I said, avoid overblouses at all cost. They look dowdy and will make you look thicker. If you're big busted, don't wear anything that falls straight from the bust. And don't, I repeat, wear short skirts or bare midriffs.

Q. Anything else you'd like to add?

A. Yes. You really can look fashionable and sexy without striving to look 20. On the other hand, some women can carry off a really off-beat look. For example, Estelle Getty, who plays Sophia on "The Golden Girls," looks great in jeans and a rhinestone-studded jean jacket. You can have your own special style. But be sure it's yours and not the trend of the moment. And be sure you can carry it off.

ACCESSORIES

Accessories are the *indispensable* tools of fashion. With them you can look stylish, key into current trends, and create your own specific image without spending a packet on clothes that will be "out" as quickly as they were "in."

HOW TO LOOK RICH—
WITHOUT SPENDING A LOT OF MONEY

Fashion stylist Corinne Van Plaar tells women how to dress "like a million dollars" without owning designer clothes (if the classic "rich girl" image is what you seek). The secret lies in making a limited investment in classic accessories: Every woman should have two pearl necklaces, one long and one short, Corinne advises. (No one will quibble if yours are good copies or the real thing.) A white or cream-colored silk blouse is another expensive-looking wardrobe essential, according to Corinne. (Here we'll call it an accessory.) With a well-tailored skirt or pair of pants, you'll always look well-dressed. Also useful is a tailored white shirt for the times when you wish to look ready for business. Corinne adds to these recommendations a list of accessories from which you might choose one or two identifiably pricey and luxurious items to further enhance your "rich girl" image:

✔ a snakeskin handbag

✔ a lizard belt

✔ a cashmere sweater

✔ a Hermes scarf

✔ a shoulder bag in creamy taupe or saddle brown leather—even good faux ("fake" in ordinary language) crocodile is acceptable, says Corinne, as are good faux jewels.

HOW TO LOOK CLASSIC—YET A LITTLE OFFBEAT

If you love classic clothes and "class" accessories but have a craving for the new and outlandish as well, you can satisfy the offbeat in your nature by putting together the classic with something a little "wild and woolly"—a tiger-skin printed scarf, an African bracelet, rhinestone-studded hair combs, fake jewel earrings, a handcrafted necklace. A few more hot tips from fashion stylist Corinne Van Plaar: Tuck a lacy

The Effect a Hat Had on Harriet

My friend Harriet tells the story of a hat she found on a construction site, a hat that suited her image like no other she ever had. "There it was, behind a plywood board," she says. "Black, high-domed, with a brim, and *covered* with dirt. I could not resist rescuing it, and you know, from the moment I popped that hat on my head (she first washed it), I felt safe under it. Safe and outrageous. I took to carrying a walking stick to complete the effect. I figured out a way of pulling my hair up and tucking it into the hatband. I know I looked a little witchy and eccentric, but wearing that hat always raised my spirits. That was a good time in my life, and I can't help thinking the hat had something to do with making it all happen."

antique handkerchief into the breast pocket of a blazer, top off a classic trench coat with an antique Stetson, and remember, a man-sized Timex is more interesting than a copy of an expensive woman's style.

A WORD ABOUT HANDBAGS, SHOES, AND STOCKINGS

Aunt Myrtle always said you could look well-dressed if your handbag and shoes looked good, no matter what else you wore. Though the small pouches and rigid mailboxlike handbags with double handles that Aunt Myrtle wore in her day are definitely out of date now, she had the right idea. Go for a large pouch shoulder bag for every day or an African-style basket with long leather handles or a handsome backpack, like the purple leather one my friend Jeanne wears. When you're not taking the quality-leather bag Corinne suggested you use for special occasions, you can carry a clutch in some less-expensive material such as velour or even a good-looking vinyl.

Put money into shoes, especially if you have bad feet. (As my friend Ellen says, "Forget wrinkles, the feet are the first to go.") Don't wear Red Cross shoes or Dr. Scholl's: They are a tip-off that you're over the hill. Search for the perfect shoe—in fit, comfort, and style, like you would hunt for a good buy in real estate. Then stay with that shoe season after season. The Calvin Klein shoes I wear fit as though they were made just for me. They make my feet feel fine, yet look spiffy. And they're actually cheaper than the dreadful looking "orthopedic" shoes I bought one season when my flat feet finally caved in. Wear a good pair of jogging or sport walking shoes to and from work and on long walking jaunts, carrying your good shoes in your bag.

Don't wear high-heeled shoes if they're uncomfortable. Wear flats or, better yet, a little heel, but don't give in to "old lady shoes" unless your doctor prescribes them.

Wear sheer stockings: black, taupe, gray, beige, tan, wine, or brown—coordinated with your shoes, skirt, or pants. Wear heavy, tweedy hose only if a country look is your intention. Novelty hosiery is fun sometimes, but beware of bright colors and excessively patterned types, especially if your legs aren't all that wonderful.

TAKING IT ON THE ROAD

So you're going to travel. How do you take your look "on the road"? Again, work with Lawson's Law of Elementary Fashion. For a short trip think in terms of your *three colors* and separates that combine into at least six combinations. It is unlikely that you'll be with the same people over and over again, so certain looks can be repeated often. Dark cotton knits are dandy to travel with year-round. They don't wrinkle. They can be washed. They can be dressed up or down with accessories. I travel with black cotton knits. A mid-calf-length skirt, pants, and a tunic are central to my traveling gear. I carry a few bracelets and earrings in a

Ten Packing Tips

1. Before you start packing, set everything out that you are thinking of taking. Then put half of it away. Put more away. Take as little as possible with you. Pack in a suitcase that meets the "carry-on" requirements on a plane, and use a shoulder bag (wear an African straw one) to carry extras, like your toilet kit or hair dryer.

2. Keep your traveling wardrobe to three or four colors: a background color like black and two others, say red and white, and maybe a fourth that harmonizes, like gray. These are the colors I take (well, these are the colors I live with). They enable me to mix and match a few clothes and accessories into an extended travel—and everyday— wardrobe. Basic to my travel wardrobe is a black dress, black skirt, and black pants, a red jacket, a black tunic top (which can double as a bathrobe and even as a sleep

shirt), a red and a black sweater, a black and red top, black dress shoes, and gray sweats and gray running shoes. If it's winter, I take a gray and white tweed coat, a red plastic raincoat, a muffler, and warm socks. If it's summer or if I'm going to a warm climate, I add a black bathing suit, black shorts, white shorts, red gym shorts for running, a couple of white T-shirts, and red plastic beach sandals.

3. Pack knits whenever possible—cotton, wool, or blends. I wear cotton knits—black, red, white, sometimes gray—year-round. They wash easily and wrinkles hang out. You roll them up to pack them.

4. Take small accessories: earrings, bracelets, belts, and scarves to change the look of a *very* few garments. I take a black and a white bone bracelet and a black and white Sonia Rykiel scarf.

baggie and take along a scarf or two—to dress up or dress down these few items. In the winter I add silk long johns and turtlenecks (ordered from the L. L. Bean catalog) for extra warmth. I also take a heavy black wool sweater, wool socks (and silk socks)—they're very warm—a large, bright red wool scarf, a black knit hat, and a fold-up, brimmed, black rainhat. Everything fits in a gray carry-on bag. I never have to wait for luggage, so it's never lost.

5. Pack small items—stockings and socks in shoes; shoes, sandals, and lingerie into the far reaches of suitcase corners. Put scarves and jewelry in a flat handbag—the only kind to pack.

6. Roll everything that's small, or that can be rolled, like a cotton knit skirt. Anything packed flat that wrinkles, like a shirt, should be stuffed with tissue paper and wrapped in plastic to prevent wrinkles and creases.

7. Before you shower, hang as many things in the bathroom as you can to steam out signs of packing. After your shower, hang longer things from the shower rail to take advantage of the lingering steam.

8. Invest in one of those hand-held steamers that looks like a mini-vacuum cleaner. Run it inside and outside of each garment that needs pressing when you take it out of the suitcase.

9. As soon as you return from your travels, make a note of any toiletries or cosmetics that need to be replaced for the next trip and keep them in your toilet kit. Don't wait until you have a spur-of-the-moment invitation to go somewhere, and no time to replenish your supplies.

10. When you're packing to come home from your vacation, jot down what you actually wore. Also write down what you didn't wear. Label the list by the place you visited, the date, and how long you stayed, i.e., West Palm Beach, Thanksgiving 1984—4 days. Keep these notes in your suitcase so you have them the next time you pack. (I have several notes labeled Wellfleet, Cape Cod; West Gardiner, Maine; Los Angeles, etc.) I've got my packing down to a science.

When you pack:

✔ No matter where you are going, try to pack in a carry-on bag. Don't put yourself through the hassle of lost luggage.

✔ Carry packets of Woolite to wash clothes as you need them.

✔ To save space, pack small items—belts, socks, and jewelry—inside shoes.

✔ Carry a large shoulder bag for day (great for day trips), a small clutch for night.

✔ If you are traveling from one climate to another, take clothes that can be layered rather than complete wardrobe changes. It is easier to pack a couple of sweaters and long underwear than a heavy coat.

✔ Pack a rain poncho in khaki or some unobtrusive color—takes up less space than a raincoat and goes with anything.

✔ Black sweatpants are great to travel in. They don't wrinkle. They're comfortable and if you're trim, they usually look good.

Chapter 7

SEX, SLEEP, SCENT & OTHER REJUVENATORS

As I write this chapter, Christmas is less than three days away (with most of our presents still unwrapped and a few to be chosen), and I am climbing the wall. I am also exhausted. In Anne Morrow Lindbergh's *Gift from the Sea* (New York: Random House, 1955), she writes, "I believe most people are aware of periods in their lives when they seem to be 'in grace' and other periods when they feel 'out of grace' even though they may use different words to describe these conditions." These days I am out of grace. What comforts me is the knowledge that our bodies have tremendous restorative powers. With two good nights' sleep in a row, great sex (well, even good sex), proper food, exercise, correct breathing, meditation (let us not forget silence), and any one of a number of other rejuvenating techniques, I'll be back "in grace" sooner than would seem possible right now.

SEX THAT SOOTHES JANGLED NERVES

Sexual release is a natural tranquilizer; it soothes jangled nerves and leaves you feeling relaxed. For those lucky enough to have an ongoing sexual relationship with a lover, sexual activity is a pleasurable and effective way to reduce tension and anxiety. But lack of a regular sexual partner shouldn't keep you from having sex. Masturbation is also a perfectly normal way to loosen up, relax, and enjoy yourself.

Well and good, but we all know about sexual snags that crop up in mid-life: the monotony of the long-term relationship, worries about losing our looks, changing physical responses and priorities, menopausal myths, and the masturbation taboo. For some expert advice on these dilemmas, I spoke with two New York City sex therapists: Dagmar O'Connor, Ph.D., director of the Sex Therapy Program, Department of Psychiatry, St. Luke's-Roosevelt Hospital Center; and Sheila Jackman, Ph.D., director of Human Sexuality, Hospital of Albert Einstein College of Medicine.

OH, NOT NOW

After you've lived with someone many years, sex can become (let us admit it!) monotonous. Familiarity breeds ennui, sexiness toward your partner subsides and excuses arise: "He doesn't turn me on," "My body has changed," "His body has changed," "I'm too tired," "I'm too busy," "We've been doing *that* forever." Still, Dr. O'Connor (author of *How to Make Love to the Same Person for the Rest of Your Life: And Still Love It* [New York: Doubleday & Company, 1985]), defends marriage. "Even though we turn ourself off in marriage, lifelong committed sex can be more thrilling, more varied, and more satisfying. It's possible for couples who have been together a long time to renew sexual energy through techniques and exercises." For one thing, Dr. O'Connor suggests reviving adolescent fantasies: Imagine people making love behind drawn window curtains; mentally undress people that you meet. And instead of watching television at night, take a brisk walk together. It's possible to add elements of seduction that re-create the thrill and adventure of conquest.

Here are a few ways that can help us rediscover our sexual feelings:

✔ For five minutes each day, get undressed and look yourself over head to toe in front of a full-length mirror. Focus on what you find attractive.

✔ Leave your pajamas and nightgown in the bureau and sleep together in the nude. If you both agree, make a deal that either of you can wake the other up. Ask for what you like. Focus on your own sexual feelings and sensations, not your partner's.

✔ One evening a week on the way home from work, pick up a bottle of wine and two sandwiches to go, and take each other to bed. Don't turn on the TV. Do turn the phone off. For the next three or four hours, just eat and drink and fool around.

✔ If you are alone on the street, stop and kiss each other right there.

Most women talk about the loss of sexual spontaneity in long-term relationships. However, Dr. O'Connor explains, sex rarely begins at the height of passion but rather with a relaxed appreciation of each other's bodies.

Dr. O'Connor says that "staying in shape physically is a prime way to get the juices going. Swimming or taking an exercise class helps you appreciate your body's strength and liveliness."

Certainly women in mid-life (and often much earlier) talk about losing their looks and becoming dissatisfied with their bodies. "Disliking your body when you're having sex is like going to a party in a dress you don't like," says Dr. O'Connor. "And if you feel this way in mid-life, how are you going to feel when you're 72?" In general, women are embarrassed about their bodies and can endlessly catalog each sag and crease, each blemish and bulge. "In my 12 years as a sex therapist, I've only met four women who were pleased with their bodies," says Dr. Jackman. "If you're uncomfortable with your body or your partner's body, you won't feel sexy," says Dr. O'Connor. Dr. Jackman offers a remedy that is especially useful for midlife women:

Stand naked in a dimly lit room and visualize the way you want to look. How would you hold your body? How would you move? When you're with other people, hold yourself and move as if you were your idealized self. Even though you're faking it, you'll elicit positive responses: "You look terrific. Have you cut your hair? Have you lost weight?" These reactions from other people—even though you're faking it—will make you feel sexier.

Men in mid-life worry about their changing responses. At around 40, when a man needs more tactile stimulation to get a full erection, he may blame his partner. ("How come *you're* not turning me on anymore?") Then, blaming ourselves, we trigger a cycle of dysfunction. Delays are not catastrophic because, as Dr. O'Connor points out, "perhaps most middle-aged men take longer to reach orgasm and to become rearoused after orgasm, but the delay is only one of minutes or hours—not days or weeks."

MYTHS ABOUT MENOPAUSE AND SEX

When women reach menopause, this often marks the beginning of more relaxed and sensitive sex, but grim expectations can become self-fulfilling prophecies. A 51-year-old woman told Dr. O'Connor that "as I expected, my sex drive dropped off right after menopause." And so it did—in her case. After menopause some women complain of physical discomfort during sex. The thinning of the vaginal walls can cause dryness. Here again, fear of discomfort can cause a tightening of the muscle around the vagina. Says Dr. O'Connor, "Vaginal exercises—stretching, putting some fingers inside the vagina, using the speculum—gives a woman a sense of owning her own genitals. Knowing the vagina is not a fragile organ often relieves discomfort. If you're comfortable with vaginal gels, then you will also lubricate naturally." When Dr. Jackman, who lectures frequently on menopause, speaks of postmenopausal women who do lubricate naturally, women invariably come up after the lecture and tell her things like: "I'm glad you said that about getting wet. I had thought I was dried up like a prune, but when I had sex with my lover, I'd get wetter than when I was 17 years old."

THE FANTASY TURN-ON

Sexual fantasies are a great way to increase arousal, but if you're uneasy about fantasies (or don't think you fantasize at all), Dr. Jackman would urge you to read Nancy Friday's *My Secret Garden* (New York: Pocket Books, 1983) and *Forbidden Flowers* (New York: Pocket Books, 1982). Don't worry if you fantasize about the "wrong" person; unfaithfulness in your head is perfectly normal and a way to make your sex life more fulfilling. In fantasies, Dr. Jackman explains, anything goes. Just make sure you include the senses—sight, smell, touch, and hearing.

THE PRIORITY PROBLEM IN MID-LIFE

According to Dr. Jackman, women mostly allow work, family, shopping—anything—to interfere with sex. Not so for men. Business may be terrible she says, but a man can push his business problems aside for sex because he knows sex makes him feel good. (True, admits Dr. Jackman, some of us—under 40 or over 40—have sexual appetites like men. The range of the normal libido is enormous. "I work with a 55-year-old woman who talks about sex with the passion of an 18-year-old," says Dr. Jackman.)

OH, BUT MOTHER SAID NO!

According to both Dr. O'Connor and Dr. Jackman, you can make love to yourself. Both men and women who are comfortable about masturbating know masturbation is about energy release and relief of tension. "That release may take only three minutes and sometimes you don't want to interact with anyone," says Dr. Jackman. "While some religions teach that masturbation's wrong, I think God approves. The real problem is that women don't hook up pelvic tension and anxiety with sexual arousal." Although most women like to think sex is an expression of love between two people, sex is the expression of more than one emotion. Sometimes it's the satisfaction of a simple bodily need. How you make love and with whom is your personal signature and an expression of who you are.

SHAPE UP YOUR SLEEP HABITS AND FEEL BETTER

Until a year ago I was a morning person ("lark") who slept solidly from 11:00 P.M. until 7:00 A.M. Then, when major stresses appeared in my life—a family illness coinciding with a particularly difficult book assignment—I began to have difficulty falling—and staying—asleep. Each day I worried that I'd never sleep again. I snapped at everyone and yawned constantly. Of course, I never looked worse, since nothing hinders your appearance like a poor night's sleep. Fortunately, several years earlier I had researched and written an article on insomnia. I knew sleep problems often begin in mid-life, just when we're looking for all the beauty benefits we can get. After two weeks of snapping and yawning, I asked myself if I should consult a sleep specialist—or try for a home-cure. In the last ten years the country's 5 sleep centers have proliferated to over 100 centers and my files were bulging with their research. Why not apply their techniques of curing insomnia to myself? If I didn't sleep better after two weeks, I'd consider a sleep specialist.

First, I thought about my lifelong sleep habits. No longer an eight-hour sleeper, I knew why. Changes in the length and depth of sleep can vary from time to time in everyone's life and those changes are normal. Wilse Webb, M.D., director of the Sleep Laboratory at the University of Florida, points out the vast range of sleep requirements: "Some people have short sleep needs and some have long sleep needs. There's about a four-hour range in adults in terms of their natural sleep links and it doesn't make them any smarter or any duller. Let them respond to their differences instead of cramming them into a procrustean bed called eight hours."

PRACTICE WHAT SLEEP RESEARCHERS CALL "SLEEP HYGIENE"

"We don't put people in the sleep lab until they've shaped up their habits," says Quentin Registein, M.D., psychiatrist and director of the Sleep Laboratory at Peter Brigham Woman's Hospital, Boston, and author of *Sound Sleep* (New York: Simon & Schuster, 1980). During this stressful period, I had in fact fallen into slipshod sleep habits: editing articles until 1:00 or 2:00 A.M. or watching late-night television. Any sleep specialist would have told me to establish a before-bedtime ritual: a hot bath and dull book. They would have told me to work in the living room instead of the bedroom (to associate the bed with sleep instead of tossing and turning) and to get out of bed and read if I woke up instead of lying there fretting.

A LOUD NO TO BARBITURATES

Maybe my family doctor would have prescribed sleeping medication, but I've never taken pills and I didn't want to start. I realized that my insomnia was most likely due to stress or a normal change in sleep patterns. I had no need for sleeping pills. They were not for me. I can recite a litany of their drawbacks. If you take sleeping pills for more than a week or two, you need a greater dose to achieve the effects of the original dose. The longer you stay on pills, the harder it is to stop. What's more, sleeping pills distort your sense of time and you could accidentally take a fatal dose. Sleeping pills also alter normal brain activity, and the natural stages of sleep are skipped or shortened. A shortened REM cycle (the dreaming stage) can produce terrifying nightmares when you stop the medication. Anthony Kales, M.D., psychiatrist and director of the sleep laboratory at Hershey Medical Center, Hershey, Pennsylvania, points out, "The medication is taken in increasingly larger and larger doses and markedly disrupts the sleep stages, primarily decreasing the rapid eye movement or dreaming sleep." Besides, sleeping pills leave you with an all-morning hangover—no asset when you need to be alert. When pills stop working on any level (but you *must* have them), you're hooked. (Unfortunately the sleeping pill habit is most established in older people who don't realize that the older you get the less sleep you need. Instead of enjoying the extra time awake, they panic and pester their doctor for sleeping pills.)

INSTEAD OF PANICKING, USE THE SLEEPLESS HOURS CONSTRUCTIVELY

My friend Kay loves the privacy of being up alone at night. When she wakes up in the middle of the night, she reads, cleans closets, writes letters, balances her checkbook, and watches old Katharine Hepburn/Spencer Tracy movies on television. She says, "I enjoy insomnia now that I've learned to deal with it." And I recalled a television program on sleep in which the interviewer asked a one-hour-a-night sleeper what she did in that spare time. She replied:

> I don't have enough spare time—oh—I've forgotten what that word means. I'm always writing or reading or painting or sewing or knitting or crocheting. I never feel tired. I feel physically tired. My legs and arms and body feel tired, but not my head. No, I'm always alert. Sleep eight hours a night? Well, it would be a bit cheaper because I have to burn electricity during the night. That's the only reason. No, I don't see any reason to want to sleep. I think it's a frightful waste of time. I get so much done.

DO YOU SMOKE? QUIT

Tobacco was not the cause of my insomnia. I had never smoked. Heavy smokers generally have a harder time falling asleep and are light sleepers. They also experience more reduced amounts of REM sleep than nonsmokers. Studies of former smokers have found that after they quit they were able to fall asleep faster and sleep longer with fewer awakenings. Their REM sleep returned, too.

NO MORE MORNING COFFEE

Having already given up all caffeine drinks after lunch, I then gave up my caffeinated cup for decaffeinated at breakfast. Coffee consumed at bedtime generally delays falling asleep and increases the number of awakenings. Even though peak stimulation occurs two to four hours after drinking coffee, its effects trouble some people and insomniacs should avoid caffeine at all times. Michael Thorpy, M.D., director of the Sleep-Wake Disorders Center, Montefiore Hospital, New York, says:

Caffeine is one of the few things that have been shown to make a significant difference. The closer to the sleep period, the more likely caffeine has an effect. We recommend that people stop taking caffeine-containing drinks after noon because of the general increased stimulation. That increased stimulation, activity, and arousal may persist after the caffeine effects have gone. I think all insomniacs should avoid any caffeinated drink.

Dr. Registein feels even more strongly: "If you drink more than three cups in a day, you can be in a stuporous state when you awaken."

NO MORE ALCOHOL WITH DINNER OR AFTER

I rarely drink, but if I do, I fall asleep quickly, then sleep fitfully. Alcohol helps you relax but the initial part of REM sleep is usually delayed, and subsequent episodes are shortened. Total REM sleep may be reduced as much as 60 percent.

PLAY SLEEP GAMES

If you wake up in the middle of the night, play sleep games. Rhyming is a good one. Start with a root sound like "atch" and then rhyme it with catch, hatch, latch, and so on. I can bore myself into sleep by counting sheep. This strategy works by distracting the brain with soothing repetition.

YOU NEED A COMFORTABLE BED AND BEDROOM

Lumpy mattress? Adequate covers? Proper pillow? If you have a husband who likes more blankets than you, consider an electric blanket with two sets of controls. Check the temperature in the room. If the place you live in is noisy, try earplugs. If your mattress is uncomfortable, get a new one.

TAKE A NAP

Half the people in the world are daily nappers. After all, the afternoon siesta is indigenous to life in the tropics and subtropics. In our society, those who can nap do so—or should. If you are one of those who boasts, "I *never* sleep in the daytime," maybe you should reconsider. Studies reveal that body rhythms drop to a low at about 2:00 P.M., and that's why our limbs grow leaden and our eyelids heavy. "If you're a siesta person, then you must be a siesta person seven days a week," says

How to Choose the Best Bedding

The Mattress

The ideal sleep environment is a darkened room with little or no noise, a temperature ranging between 64 and 68°F, and a firm, back-supporting mattress that is less than eight to ten years old. Robert G. Addison, M.D., director of the center for pain studies at the Rehabilitation Institute of Chicago, described the mattress problem and its solution.

All night long as you sleep on a too-soft or too-hard bed, your muscles are working overtime to align your spine. It's no coincidence that many people wake up in the morning with a backache. They haven't given those muscles any time off to rest. No bed is perfectly suited to everyone because we're all built differently and we have different needs for support. Two general rules seem to prevail:

✔ An ideal mattress should hold the spine as closely as possible to a position you would assume while standing with good posture.

✔ This position should be held in a way that distributes your body weight evenly with no one part of the body being pressured more than another.

These are two pretty basic requirements, actually, but these requirements can get lost in the shuffle when it comes time to buy a mattress from a store. Most stores carry between one and five brands of bedding, each coming in three to seven different degrees of firmness. Let your comfort be your guide. Give a mattress a good ten-minute test run before even thinking about buying it. And when your salesman begins to talk number of coils, listen. Coils count in terms of both durability and performance.

What about saving your old mattress with a bed board? Not a good idea, particularly if you've got a touchy back. Adjustable posture beds won't help your back either.

In the final analysis, it seems a high-quality, firm mattress supported by the box spring that was designed to go with it is best for most people, especially for those with bad backs.

The Pillow

A good pillow is as important as a good mattress. What's the best kind? Lionel Walpin, M.D., clinical director of physical medicine at Cedars/Sinai Medical Center in Los Angeles, says the type of pillow you use depends on the type of sleeper you are:

✔ Back sleepers should use a pillow that's thin and soft—but not too thin and soft. Avoid the type of pillow that forces you to scrunch up your neck and shoulders to keep the pillow in place (causing tension to neck and shoulder muscles).

✔ Side sleepers with narrow shoulders should also use a thin pillow. Side sleepers with broad shoulders should choose a thicker model.

✔ Choose a pillow that discourages you from sleeping on your stomach, a sleeping posture that puts pressure on your jaw and irritates neck muscles.

✔ Choose a pillow that doesn't slide or roll away.

✔ Choose a pillow that eliminates the need to place your arm or hand under the pillow. Sleeping this way can cause pinched nerves in the elbow or wrist.

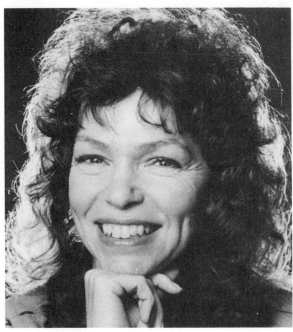

Gretchen Cryer

Dr. Registein. "You can't go back and forth. The consistency is more important than the pattern. Look at the navy. Sailors stand two four-hour watches so they work from 8:00 A.M. until noon and then 8:00 P.M. until midnight. They sleep twice daily under these circumstances. No problem as long as you do the same thing all the time."

The Pros and Cons of Napping

Noted nappers include Winston Churchill, Chou En-lai, Harry S. Truman, Henry Kissinger, Thomas Edison, John F. Kennedy. Does this mean that men alone are born with the gift of enjoying the midday snooze? Not at all. Barbara Walters naps. So does Gretchen Cryer, an actress and composer in her fifties (*I'm Getting My Act Together and Taking It on the Road*). She naps during ten-minute rehearsal breaks. And my friend Martha, a free-lance writer, enthusiastically praises naps:

> There isn't a single day when I can't nap for a few minutes. When I wake up, I can work or play into the deep of night. I've always been able to fall asleep immediately, preferably around two in the afternoon, but if that's inconvenient, then a little later or a little earlier. I have a way of taking naps for ten minutes, anywhere at all. I just shut my eyes and imagine that I'm lying on the beach listening to the ocean waves.

Another friend, Joan, an advertising executive/dynamo, naps for an energy jolt. Her secretary screens calls while Joan knocks off for a five-minute nap after lunch. Joan says she gets twice as much done because of her nap habit.

Should *You* Nap?

Where do *you* stand on lying down in the middle of the day? Your yes or no answers to the following informal quiz will give you a clue:

		YES	NO
1.	Do you awaken from your nap bright-eyed and refreshed?	☐	☐
2.	Is your vigor renewed?	☐	☐
3.	Does a nap sweep the cobwebs from your brain?	☐	☐
4.	Can you switch sleep on and off at will?	☐	☐
5.	Can you doze off whether you're tired or not?	☐	☐
6.	Do you enjoy napping?	☐	☐
7.	Do you nap a minute or so to an hour at most?	☐	☐
8.	Do you nap as a daytime break from tension and stress (in addition to a full six to eight hours of sleep at night)?	☐	☐
9.	Does the mere process of relaxing elevate your mood?	☐	☐
10.	Does your performance improve when you awake from your nap?	☐	☐
11.	Do you nap to fight fatigue?	☐	☐
12.	Do you nap to make up for lost nighttime rest?	☐	☐
13.	Do you usually fall into a sound sleep that may last 1½ hours? (A REM sleep is difficult to pull out of.)	☐	☐
14.	Do you often feel bushed and out of sorts when you wake up with (as my friend Betty says) "sweaters on your teeth"?	☐	☐

If you answered yes to the first ten questions, you are an "appetitive" napper. A midday snooze won't disturb your nighttime sleep in the least. If you answered no to the first ten questions and yes to the last four, you are a "replacement" napper. Naps cut into your nighttime sleep, so you'd best concentrate on that. How you sleep at night determines whether daytime napping will be restorative or not. Although most of us could improve our daytime alertness by getting a little more sleep at night, those with chronic insomnia may have a bad reaction to a daytime nap because it will interfere with an already erratic sleep pattern. Most sleep experts believe insomniacs should concentrate on falling asleep at bedtime. When you nap to *replace* sleep lost the night before, you reach a deep stage of sleep. That's why you wake up groggy.

How to Doze Off If You Want to Nap

Don't feel guilty about napping. Afternoon drowsiness is part of our innate rhythms, urging us to take a break from stress. If you've had a good night's sleep, you'll sleep less than a half hour and you won't be wasting time.

Try these relaxation exercises, alternately tensing and releasing one part of your body at a time: first your feet, then your legs, arms, stomach, and so forth, until you've reached your neck and finally your face. Breathe deeply to bring on drowsiness. Take slow, deep breaths in a series of three, exhaling fully after each. At the end of the third exhalation, hold your breath as long as possible. Then repeat the series. After five to eight of them, you'll want to breathe normally. By then you should be relaxed and ready to sleep.

Visualize something pleasant that you've enjoyed or are looking forward to—a favorite spot in the country, a beach romp, or your next vacation. Take your mind off the unpleasant or ordinary to help you relax.

If you have trouble uncluttering your mind of a whole series of overwhelming problems, select one and concentrate on it carefully, breaking it down into all its parts and examining each fact. Don't allow yourself to think of any of the other problems, but stick to only the one you've chosen.

Rest even if you don't sleep. Close your office door if you have one, and put your feet up. (When my friend Sue worked on a magazine, she had her own office but not the authority to close her door. After lunch, she'd go up to the nurse's station and ask, "May I lie down? I have a dreadful headache." After closing her eyes for ten minutes, she was recharged.) Breaking away from a stressful environment for only a moment or two can do wonders to erase frown lines and lift sagging spirits.

Keep your nap under an hour. If you sleep longer, your sleep pattern will go askew.

EXERCISE DAILY FOR A HALF HOUR IN THE LATE AFTERNOON OR EARLY EVENING

My life was so hectic that I got sloppy about exercise. I let my health club membership lapse so it was easy to make excuses. Vowing a new era of self-discipline, I renewed my membership and swam every day at 8:00 A.M. I didn't notice much change in my sleep habits—for a good reason. Early morning exercise has no effect on sleep at night, according to Arthur J. Sprelman, Ph.D., director, Sleep Disorders Center—the College of New York. So it looks like the best time to exercise (at least to improve sleep) is between 4:00 and 8:00 P.M. I still swim at 8:00 A.M. because I don't have time later in the day.

How Exercise Affects the Quality of Your Sleep

Exercise exhausts your muscles. And it's physical exhaustion that introduces you to stage one of the sleep cycle—a kind of semiconsciousness that leads to progressively deeper stages of sleep, culminating in what doctors consider the all-important dream state.

There is no way to skip stages. What happens is that the rhythm of your sleep changes so you spend relatively more time in a phase that sleep researchers call slow wave sleep, or SWS. SWS is a very deep form of sleep that is also the most restorative, especially to the physical body. Samual Dunkel, M.D., says, "Strenuous exercise for half an hour three times a week increases SWS, but this should not be done too close to sleep because after strenuous exercise the body is very stimulated. Several hours before bedtime is fine."

Will you sleep longer if you exercise? If you take up exercise, you may sleep less. "It's been my experience," says Allan Ryan, M.D., editor-in-chief of the *Physician and Sports Medicine,* "that exercise, if anything, reduces the amount of time people need to spend in bed by helping them to fall asleep in the first place."

DRINK A WARM GLASS OF MILK AT BEDTIME

L-tryptophan is a tranquilizing amino acid compound that seems to be effective in helping people (including the actress Bernadette Peters) fall asleep without distorting sleep stages or causing side effects. Amino acids, as you probably know, are the basic building blocks of protein, and L-tryptophan is contained in protein-rich foods such as milk, eggs, almost any meat, certain fish such as salmon or bluefish, and dairy products, especially cottage cheese. Or you can take two 500-milligram tablets.

CURING OTHER SLEEP PROBLEMS WITH CHRONOTHERAPY

As any insomniac will tell you, you want to discuss your fatigue and despair with everyone. (Of course, people who sleep well find the topic boring, so don't even try to engage them in a discussion of sleeplessness and crankiness.) During my bout with insomnia (which, incidentally, ceased when my book was finished on time and I fine-tuned my habits), I found a soul mate in my friend Nancy, the night owl. Nancy is not your everyday night person but a night person with "delayed sleep phase syndrome," resulting from a dysfunction of her circadian rhythms. Even if Nancy is bone-tired, she cannot fall asleep before 4:00 A.M. Once asleep, she sleeps eight hours. When Nancy sleeps until noon (on vacations and weekends), she wakes refreshed, but her nine-to-five job (more or less) requires a punctual arrival. Nancy can hardly manage that: She sets her alarm for 7:00 and on what might be as little as three hours' sleep, arrives at her office half-dazed, eyes swollen, and disposition surly. So she functions poorly for half her workday. Nancy can change her sleep pattern by shifting her daily sleep cycle until it corresponds to a cycle that meshes with the demands of a nine-to-five job. In chronotherapy, Nancy would reset her biological clock by going to bed three hours later every day until her cycle advanced to a conventional bedtime. (For instance, the first day she'd go to sleep at 7:00 A.M. and sleep eight hours; the second day, she'd go to sleep at 10:00 A.M. and sleep eight hours.) After about a week, Nancy would "move entirely around the clock" until she trained herself to the schedule that would work best for her both socially and professionally. People like Nancy are like clocks that you can reset only by moving the hands forward, not backward.

WHERE TO FIND CENTERS FOR SLEEP DISORDERS

If *your* sleep problems persist, you may want to go to a sleep laboratory. The doctors will ask for details of your medical history, the

---

How to Face Life When You Awaken

If you look like an apparition in the morning (I can barely look at myself in the mirror no matter how well I've slept), these three morning pickups will perk you up and get you off to a good start:

1. Get physical (the cure for everything). Good circulation is an important factor in making yourself feel and look good in the morning. By doing some simple stretching routines or aerobics, you'll improve your blood flow.

2. There's nothing like water to get your circulatory system going at full speed. Stimulate your skin by rinsing your face alternately with warm, then cool, water. Drinking water also will help replenish the body fluids you've lost overnight (which makes you feel sluggish).

3. Instead of a breakfast packed with lots of calories or no breakfast at all, try this heavenly midlife health shake:

Heavenly Midlife Health Shake

1 cup orange juice
1 small banana
¼ cup plain yogurt
⅛ teaspoon ground nutmeg

Place all ingredients in a blender, and whirl until smooth.
Yield: 1 glass.

details of your sleeping habits, and the temperature of your bedroom. They'll find out if depression or medical problems are disturbing your sleep, and they'll prescribe a treatment suitable for your particular problem. For accreditation status and further information, write to the Association of Sleep Disorders Center, P.O. Box 2604, Del Mar, CA 92014.

USE SCENT TO RELAX AS WELL AS ATTRACT

Wear perfume. Light fragrant oil lamps and French candles. Make potpourris. Slip sachets into your bureau drawers. Collect pungent flowers. Scent your sheets. Take a heady bubble bath. Keep the windows open. Cook with herbs. Keep pots or vases of sweet-smelling flowers in your house.

We underestimate the powers of scent. Oh, we've all fretted over what perfume would make us alluring, but sometimes the everyday smells pass us by. (Notice how the word smell is not quite as alluring as perfume or scent.) Actually our response is instinctive and immediate: Months or years later, a particular smell will activate old memories, and past events will suddenly enter our awareness. Sometimes we do it on purpose. My friend Annie, for instance, carries a tiny bottle of spiced apple fragrance, which she'll sniff a minute or two to evoke memories of the Virginia farm of her childhood. But apricots bring back memories of my childhood in southern California (we lived near a grove of apricot trees), which accounts for my addiction to apricot soap and shampoo. And jasmine reminds me of adolescent grapplings in various parked convertibles on Hollywood's fragrant Mulholland Drive. (A friend, who also remembers Mulholland Drive, once planted jasmine under her bedroom window to heal a failing marriage. The marriage failed anyway.)

We've all got a memory storehouse containing a thousand smells, the release of which (like the taste of Proust's *Madeleine*) brings back events long forgotten by our conscious minds. What's surprising to me is that we are more likely to react violently to a smell than to a sight or a sound; not surprisingly, some people are more sensitive to odors than others. "Smell is our strongest sense," says Susan Schiffman, Ph.D., scent researcher and associate professor at the Department of Psychiatry, Duke University. "A pleasant, evocative fragrance gives us an overall sense of well-being."

I'm filled with well-being from Fracas, a perfume I've worn for 15 years. I splash it on several times a day for a lift, and I'm not really sure if its floral, almost tropical, scent reminds me of an attractive man I once met in Paris or if its oils contain stimulating properties. I do know that as Tiffany's cheered up Holly Golightly *(Breakfast at Tiffany's),* so Caswell-Massey, New York's oldest and sweetest-smelling pharmacy, cheers me.

I'll drop into C.M. every now and then for an orgy of scent—jasmine, honeysuckle, wisteria, tea rose, bergamot, neroli....You name a fragrance, I've got a memory.

Right now, according to Annette Green, executive director, Fragrance Foundation, major cosmetics companies are testing "health maintenance" fragrances that will one day reduce stress by day and induce sleep at night. And scientists in laboratories at Yale and Duke have already found that certain scents produce changes in blood pressure and other physiological responses comparable to responses to meditation. In the near future you may be able to treat your down moods through your sense of smell.

Some people are less receptive to scent than I am. My friend Jane tells me she deliberately turns down her response to smells, lest she

Make Your Own Fragrant Potpourri

Potpourri is a mixture of dried flower petals, citrus rinds, herbs, and spices that is kept in a covered jar and, when the lid is lifted, fills a room with fragrance.

To make your own potpourri, begin by gathering rose petals in the early morning. Toss them onto a table in a cool, airy place to lie until the dew has dried off; then put them in a large stone jar, sprinkling a little salt over each ½-inch layer of petals. Add to your pile of petals from morning to morning until enough roses have been gathered for your purpose. Let them stand in the jar for ten days after the last are gathered, stirring every morning. Mix together 2 tablespoons each of cloves, coarsely ground allspice, and stick cinnamon that has been broken and shredded finely with the fingers. Transfer the petals to another jar and scatter the spices in layers alternately with the petals.

Cover the jar tightly and let it stand in a dark place for three weeks, when the stock will be ready for a permanent jar. Have ready ½ tablespoon each of mace, allspice, and cloves all coarsely ground; ½ tablespoon of dried nutmeg; 1 tablespoon of stick cinnamon broken finely; 2 tablespoons of powdered orris root; add ¼ pound of dried lavender flowers. Mix all together in a bowl and proceed to fill the rose jar with alternate layers of stock and this last mixture. A few drops each of several essential oils—rose geranium, neroli, and bitter almond—should be sprinkled on the layers as you progress. Over all, pour 2 tablespoons of fine cologne or rosewater. This is sufficient to fill two 1-quart jars or one very large jar.

This potpourri should keep for years. Occasionally, various sweet things may be added—a few leaves of lemon for example. If the jar is left open 30 minutes each day, it will fill your room with a delicate, exquisite aroma.

encounter an unpleasant odor. By blunting this sense (many times stronger than taste, they say) she could be missing out on real pleasure. Smog, pollution, smoking, and congestion impair the sense of smell. However, people can train themselves to build scent memory and strengthen scent recognition.

The trend toward ordering special blends of fragrances, even making your own, is growing. The Perfumers Workshop (which you can find in Bloomingdale's, Bullocks, Robinson's, Marshall Field, and Higbee's) mixes essential oils to individual specification. And if you have $1,000 to spend, Caswell-Massey will blend essences to your special order, incorporating the perfume into a whole line: soaps, lotions, and creams. But if you don't have $1,000 to spend and you want to experiment on your own, try making this scented gem.

Lemon-Honey-Almond Oil Scented Lotion

Carefully blend equal parts (8 tablespoons each will do) of strained fresh lemon juice, honey, and almond oil in an enamel or Pyrex pan over a low flame. Remove the pan from the heat. Bottle the lotion and refrigerate it. Rub it over your body to soften the skin and give it fragrance.

ESCAPE TO THE TUB FOR A LONG, LUXURIOUS SOAK

Bath buffs, pin up your hair and go to the tub. I was a fervent shower person until New York's blackout several years ago. Taking a soothing bath by candlelight, I decided at the time, was one sensible approach to the inconvenience of an evening without electricity. So delightfully indulgent was that bath that I've been bathing instead of showering whenever I want to relax.

Baths are the ultimate luxury: accessible, private, sensual. A bath, as someone once said, is a small vacation (and much less expensive than jetting to Paris) that takes you away from family squabbles, work pressures, and kitchen chores. So leave your IOUs, your TV, and your VCR for a wonderful wallow in warm—not hot—water.

Don't forget to make your bathroom enticing. Fill it, even a small one, with flowers and plants (they love the moisture). Scent the bathwater with oils or crystals or herbs. Keep a supply of sponges, loofahs, and scented soaps by the tub. Tuck a bath pillow under your head, float flowers in the tub, play Brahms on a cassette recorder (but place it far enough away, preferably on the floor, to avoid shock!). While you're lolling, treat your eyes to some oil-saturated pads; use a natural bristle brush, a rough hand mitt, and a pumice stone (for tough spots like elbows and heels) to bring out the glow of your skin. (**Warning:** Don't make the water too hot or sit there longer than 20 minutes because your skin will dry up and you'll look like a prune.)

This is a good time to test the powers of rose and jasmine. If you're feeling jumpy, put five drops of "rose absolute" in the bath. If you're a little tired or blue, put five drops of "jasmine absolute" in the bath.

But for a sure thing, try the first three baths that I invented and the last one from aromatherapist Jeanne Rose's *Herbs and Things* (New York: Grosset & Dunlap, 1972):

Glycerine Bath

Glycerine is cheaper than bath oil (a bottle of glycerine at the drugstore can usually be bought for under a dollar). Drop a tablespoonful in your bathwater. For fragrance add rose water. (Glycerine's also nice because it keeps a ring from forming around the tub.)

Old-Fashioned Oatmeal Bath

Put four or five small portions of oatmeal tied up in squares of cheesecloth in your bath. The oatmeal will give the bathwater a milky appearance and your skin a glossy glow.

Lemon Bath

Dump a cup of freshly squeezed lemon juice into the tub. For fun wash with lemon soap. It cools your skin and soothes your nerves on a hot day and reduces oil in the skin.

Peppermint Tea Bath

Add 1 to 1½ cups of peppermint tea to one quart of boiling water. Allow the tea to stand for 30 minutes or until it's cool enough not to burn your skin. Then strain it through cheesecloth into the bathwater. This is a terrific cooler for both nerves and skin on a hot summer's day—so soothing, in fact, that it has been called the insomniac's bath.

LEARN TO MEDITATE

Meditation—another tool to take you away from the world—clears your head, calms, and refreshes. How to do it? Most relaxation techniques are variations of transcendental meditation. Try this:

✔ Get comfortable. Lean back in a chair with your feet up if you like.

✔ Breathe in slowly through your nose, then breathe out. Do this about ten times with your eyes closed while loosening your tense muscles as much as you can.

✔ As you breathe out, say "relax" or "calm" to yourself.

✔ Continue this for about two minutes, then picture in your mind a beautiful, peaceful scene. Keep yourself engrossed in the scene until you feel all the tension draining out of your body.

✔ Get up, stretch, and then loosen some of your muscles, and you will probably feel just fine. Try this when you can't sleep at night.

CUT DOWN ON ALCOHOL OR STOP DRINKING IT ALTOGETHER

Alcohol disturbs more than your sleep. In a study of 93 randomly selected women from the Irvine area in California, Dr. Isabel M. Birnbaum, a professor of psychology at the University of California, found that the amount of alcohol consumed was strongly related to mood disturbances during sobriety. Women who reduced alcohol consumption for a six-week period had significant reductions in mood disturbances, whereas those who maintained or increased alcohol consumption showed more mood disturbances at the end of six weeks. Dr. Birnbaum's conclusion: Women don't drink *because* they're depressed but *become* depressed or angry when they drink even moderate amounts of alcohol. (Besides, alcohol seriously depletes the body's reserve of stress-reducing vitamin B complex.)

A NICE CUP OF TEA WILL MAKE EVERYTHING BETTER

The tea ceremony is a civilized ritual, and most countries have their version. The Japanese have their Zen tea ceremony. The English have high tea for schoolchildren and coal miners (eggs, sausages, and beans) or afternoon tea (clotted cream, raspberry cakes, and scones), served by uniformed servants in surroundings of potted palms, cozy chintz-covered armchairs, and gleaming silver tea sets. How well I remember the gracious Lady Margery Bellamy ("Upstairs, Downstairs") pouring tea in her elegant Edwardian parlor until we lost her to the *Titanic*. Then there's my friend Eva, a stranger from England when we met in airline training school 25 years ago, who taught me the joy of tea for stress. After settling into the New York apartment we planned to share, we were robbed: our cozy nest was ransacked, and our nerves

Donna's Tranquility Cocktail

1 tablespoon bran flakes
1 tablespoon toasted wheat
   germ
1 tablespoon soy lecithin
1 tablespoon brewer's yeast
1 banana, sliced (for taste)
½ cup nonfat dry milk (for
   extra protein and calcium)
whole or skim milk

Add all ingredients except whole or skim milk to a blender. Then fill the blender with whole or skim milk, and whirl until smooth. Keep in a thermos and substitute for coffee throughout the day.

were shot. "My God, Eva, what shall we do?" I cried frantically. Eva, her brow furrowed in thought for a moment, spoke quietly: "A nice cup of tea will make everything better." I still follow Eva's formula. Every afternoon around 4 o'clock, when you could scrape me off my office floor, I'll pause for a tea break: blackberry these days. Some other soothing teas include chamomile, peppermint, spearmint, and vervain. When I want a real zinger, I drink catnip. I'm as addicted to catnip as our cat Laurence, who chews up my teabag (Lady Margery's tea was properly loose!) if he can get his grubby little paws on it.

BUILD UP A SUPPORT SYSTEM OF FAMILY AND FRIENDS

Friendship is the inexpressible comfort
of feeling safe with a person having
neither to weigh thoughts nor measure words.
George Meredith

On a par with intelligent eating, staying in shape, and the avoidance of cigarettes and alcohol is the Great Nourishing Support System. When our mothers told us to "play with our friends," they doubtlessly didn't realize how smart they were.

I knew this intuitively and through experience; now my intuition is backed up by scientific literature. It seems that people who have a close-knit network of intimate personal ties avoid disease, maintain higher levels of health, and, in general, deal more successfully with life's difficulties than people who don't. University of California public health professor S. Leonard Syme states:

> Every time I found evidence of disrupted social relationships, I found evidence of some sort of negative health outcome. And the range of disease outcome is very broad indeed. For example, people with interrupted social ties exhibit more depression, unhappiness, and loss of morale...higher mortality rates for many diseases including heart disease and cancer, higher morbidity rates for such illnesses as gastrointestinal upset, skin problems, arthritis, and headaches.

The Importance of Friendship

In a study of 4,725 residents of Alameda County in the San Francisco Bay Area, University of California public health professor S. Leonard Syme and Lisa Berkman, Ph.D., Institution for Social and Policy Studies at Yale, traced the connection between each person's social support systems and life span over a nine-year period. With few exceptions, those people who had many friends and relatives and saw them frequently lived longer than those who had fewer or saw them less frequently. Furthermore, members of religious groups had lower mortality rates than nonmembers. And it has long been known that especially close-knit religious groups like Seventh-Day Adventists and Mormons live longer, healthier lives than most of the rest of the population.

But there's an addendum to this. A cardinal rule of beauty and fitness (my own) is: Don't hang out with downbeats who sap your energy and drag you down. Sometimes you're not aware that it's happening. But think. Don't you know chronic whimperers who undermine your own good humor? Haven't you waited eagerly for a friend only to see her trudge sullenly toward you? Doesn't it place a damper on your meeting before you've even said hello? On the other hand, you know people whose élan and wit (even in the face of adversity) ignite your own humor, and you charge forth renewed in spirit after you meet. Gloominess is contagious, but so is optimism. I'm reminded of my friend Carla whose tonic personality never fails to cheer me up when I'm low—and her husband, Bob, who's fond of the expression, "Is your glass half empty or half full?" Keep your relationships with whiners and pessimists to a minimum; seek out those who like to laugh and know how to enjoy life.

Stretching for Relaxation

The Cat	The Rocker	The Rag Doll
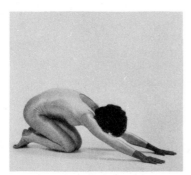	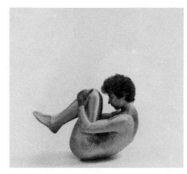	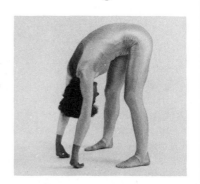

To smooth out jittery nerves in shoulders and back, get down on all paws. Arch your back right up toward the ceiling. Stretch spine forward, head toward floor. Then stretch back all the way down until you're sitting on your feet.

Rolling unwinds a coiled up spine. Lie down. Clasp your hands under your knees and roll forward and backward. Rock gently so as not to hurt any backbones on the hard floor.

Dangling takes care of nerves everywhere. Think of yourself as a floppy rag doll. Let arms droop to the floor. Swing them up and around in a great giant circle clockwise. Switch direction and do it counterclockwise a few times.

EXERCISE VIGOROUSLY

Vigorous exercise is great for frazzled nerves. By vigorous I mean exercise that gets you to "let go" completely and leaves you totally loose. Here's the story: Exercises produce the kind of relaxation that comes from the release of physical tension, a release you don't get from reading a novel in your favorite armchair. Vigorous movement means your body's circulatory system will operate at peak efficiency. Your capillaries expand during exercise so more blood can flow to the muscles. "Any kind of pleasurable physical activity—dancing or vigorous walking, for instance—makes a big difference in your breathing and emotional state," says Aileen Crow, a specialist in the Alexander Technique (a method to improve body alignment and posture). "My grandmother square danced until she was 91."

This extra physical activity uses up the negative energy that builds up in response to the stresses and strains of life. If you constantly repress day-to-day stress (and who doesn't?), exercise is one of the best ways to avoid climbing the walls. Rene Jules Dubos, Ph.D., professor at the Rockefeller Institute in New York, believes that each overreaction to stressful situations leaves the body and mind with cumulative scars that can eventually result in physical or perhaps mental disorders.

What if you're tied up in knots but you're not in the mood for vigorous exercise? You can work out those kinks by strolling in the country or even in a midtown oasis such as New York's Central Park. Relief comes quickly.

BE OPEN TO ADVICE AND PLEASURE FROM UNEXPECTED SOURCES

You will often have a good time when you least plan it, as I realized when I read a piece, "Depression Saga," from the *Playbill*. It was a story that took place during the Great Depression, in the year 1932 to be exact, about a down-and-out actor who was sitting in Central Park. An old lady sat down next to him, and soon he was telling her all his problems—no work, sickness, loss of money, and family difficulties. She dismissed all his problems with a wave of her hand. "My philosophy," she intoned, "is just to be glad you're alive." With that, she pulled a large card out of her bag and said to him, "Go to this place. Eddie Cantor, George Jessel, and lots of other people will be there. Have a good time." As she walked away, he looked at the card, and it turned out to be an invitation to the funeral of the great talent agent, William Morris. He went and had a marvelous time.

Probably you wouldn't expect to have a marvelous time if you came out of a theater one night and found it raining so hard you couldn't get a cab. Well, an actor reported that he had seen Ruth Gordon just before her death at 88 jumping up and down in a puddle like a child because she was so pleased at the rain.

I'm reminded of writer/anthropologist Ashley Montagu saying that we would all stay young if we retained the curiosity of children as we grew older. Don't be too mature.

Letting Worries Go and Making the Most of Life's Moments

Romana Kryzanowska is a former dancer and now doyenne of the studio where the Pilates Method is taught to the likes of dancers Suzanne Farrell and Jacques D'Amboise, actresses Candice Bergen and Jill Clayburgh—and plainer people like me. Romana was the prime disciple of Joseph Pilates, who devised and developed the Pilates Method over 60 years ago. The Pilates Method is a series of isotonic movements in balanced sequence.

Romana, a grandmother, refuses to let worries weigh on her. She does as much as she can to improve a bad situation on the spot and forget about it when she's away from it. "When I have hassles at the studio, I try to work them out and if I can't, I leave them there. I always walk home so I can use that time to make the transition from studio worries to the peace of my home."Romana tries to make every event as much fun as possible—even drinking a cup of tea, which she brews in a samovar and serves in paper-thin porcelain cups she bought in Chinatown. Romana, an exponent of positive living, says, "I've gone through ordeals but I worked them out and got on with living. My mother and my grandmother taught me this attitude. You can't be lazy and have a good life. You must work at life—at marriage, at friendship, at parenting, the works."

GO FOR THE BELLY LAUGH

About five years ago, when it was November in my soul, I noticed that no matter how caustic and cruel Joan Rivers's humor, she could make me laugh so hard I'd fall over. Suddenly I'd feel exhilarated instead of depressed. Why Joan Rivers had such power over me I didn't know. Then I read *Anatomy of an Illness As Perceived by the Patient* (New York: W. W. Norton, 1979) by Norman Cousins, and I began to see why. Cousins, former editor of the *Saturday Review* and now adjunct professor of medical humanities at the School of Medicine at UCLA, claimed that humor helped him recover from a degenerative spinal condition. Watching Marx brothers' movies and segments of "Candid Camera" evoked ten minutes of belly laughter and an hour of pain-free sleep. Laughter, Cousins claimed, caused the muscles of his abdomen, chest, and shoulders to contract, his heart and respiration rates to increase, and his blood pressure to dip below normal. He compared laughing to jogging.

Far-fetched? Since then, physicians have seriously researched the subject of laughter and healing. According to Dr. William Fry of Stanford University, laughter does indeed increase respiratory activity, oxygen exchange, muscular activity, and heart rate: It stimulates the cardiovascular system, sympathetic nervous system, pituitary gland, and the production of hormones called catecholamines—which in turn stimulate the brain's production of endorphins, the body's natural pain-reducing enzymes, which are chemical cousins to the opiates morphine and heroin. The production of these endorphins may cause "runner's high"—and may similarly cause "laughter's high."

A year ago I received an announcement from the Institute for the Advancement of Human Behavior about a conference on "The Healing Power of Laughter and Play." "Throughout history," the brochure read, "comedians have given us the gift of laughter. In good times and in bad, laughter has served as a 'natural healer', providing us with the sense of well-being and good health that we all need."

So it would seem that Joan Rivers in a real physiological way reduces my stress in the way that running does. My friend Griselda White attributes her enormous energy and "youthfulness" to working with babies. Doesn't that seem far-fetched? It's not. Babies and small children are funny and their humor's catching. We probably had a good sense of humor when we were babies. As babies, I've read, we all started laughing when we were 10 weeks old, usually in reaction to such sensations as bowel movements or passing gas. When we were 16 weeks old we laughed about once an hour and at 4 years we laughed about once every four minutes.

"Babies Replenish Me"

Griselda White, 52, a dancer and infant development specialist who teaches at Tufts University, accounts for her enormous energy and youthful appearance:

Babies. I work with newborn babies. Talk with them. Dance with them. Listen to them. With babies we smile as we talk and listen with waves of life-replenishing emotion. Babies shut up when there is nothing worth saying (or hearing), and they work to extract every bit of delight out of experience. Babies would agree with St. Augustine that delight orders the soul. I would add that babies order an ageless existence, and working with them I, too, am ageless.

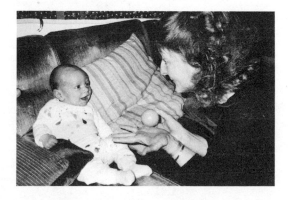

That is my only secret of youth. Of course, a little dieting, dancing, singing, and listening to or humming Brahms's Fourth Symphony helps.

Maybe I laughed a lot as a baby, but by the time I was 20, my sense of humor had lapsed. I counted on Ingmar Bergman movies to make me appear "deep," and soon I fell into thinking only serious thoughts. My dad used to say, "Why, for God's sake, don't you go to a comedy or musical?" I thought my poor old dad was just too unsophisticated while I was being ever so intellectual. (Pretentious was what I was.) Back in my Ingmar Bergman days, I hadn't lived long enough to savor life's real treats. Now that I'm middle-aged, I avoid solemn movies like poison and see comedies whenever possible. My stepchildren in their early twenties see Ingmar Bergman movies. They think I'm just too unsophisticated and (need I add!), they're ever so intellectual. At 48, I'd trade in a tear for a laugh any time.

But what if your 40-year-plus sense of humor has diminished? What if you can't make anyone laugh? Well, it doesn't matter if you're not witty. You still laugh at other people's humor. Everyone does. Even my friend Rhoda, a most solemn person who never uttered a witty word in her life, breaks into laughter if you hit the right subjects.

What if Joan Rivers or the Marx brothers or "Candid Camera" fail to amuse you? That's OK, you have your own sources of laughter. Consider, though, my dilemma. I knew Joan Rivers had laugh power over me. But we weren't friends. I couldn't call her for lunch to sneak in a laugh. At that time she didn't appear on my TV screen at the flip of a switch. Ah, but she does now. With a VCR (you have a VCR, don't you?), you can tape the people who make you laugh. They're ready to entertain you when November's in your soul. I've taped Charlie Chaplin, Woody Allen, the "Cosby Show," Johnny Carson, and Bob Hope. My latest addition to "humor" tapes is the glamorously dressed Joan Collins hawking kitchen products for Sanyo. And now I'm the goddess of mirth.

How does laughing work? According to Norman Cousins, "The most important thing...is to try to relieve the hopelessness...negative emotions—fear, hate, and rage, for example, which can weaken the body to the point where it can bring your defenses down and make you more susceptible to disease.... Love, hope, faith, laughter, and creativity are essential parts of staying well."

LISTEN TO MUSIC FOR CALMING DOWN OR PEPPING UP

Music, as I'm sure you know, is one of the oldest therapies. While you may have been surprised at the physiological effects of belly laughs and fantasy, you know full well the emotional effects of music. Maybe you can't carry a tune or play an instrument, but you've been profoundly affected by lullabies, religious music, and Christmas carols. You've shivered with patriotism to the "Star-Spangled Banner," been turned on (or repelled) by rock, and gnashed your teeth to canned music while captive to telephone hold.

How you respond to the three main elements of music—rhythm, melody, and harmony—is very personal so I won't tell you what to listen to. But, I will tell you how I learned to pep up.

In my first exercise class in New York about 15 years ago, we stretched and extended and flexed and pointed and jumped to Billy Joel's "Piano Man." Now 15 years later when I play "Piano Man" on our stereo, I'm shot with energy. Then some time after my exercise encounter with "Piano Man," I took a three-day course in "Superlearning." During the weekend, our instructor told us that music makes you concentrate. He played records—some classical, some jazz—but the one that moved me the most was Billy Joel's "Uptown Girl." For some reason "Uptown Girl" delivers me from the doldrums as "Piano Man" sends me to situps and knee bends. Billy Joel peps, but almost any hymn calms my jitters. What makes me sob are weepy Russian folk songs. What makes me stand tall is reveille and the man I march to is John Philip Sousa. Not surprisingly, a psychiatrist friend told me that psychiatric patients relax by listening to Handel's "Largo" or Bach's "Air from the Suite in D Major." And I've heard about Mozart, Bach, and Verdi's music being used as balm for depressives. So when you're about to go bonkers, try music.

KEEP YOUR PERSPECTIVE

In times of trouble, don't fall off the track. To thine own self be true. Take a lesson from the life of Mussolini's widow. Rachele Guidi met Mussolini in 1906 while working in the kitchen at his father's inn. He threatened to commit suicide if she would not marry him, but they lived together five years before the union was made legal in 1915. During il Duce's rise and reign from 1922 to 1943, Donna Rachele remained at home, keeping house and rearing their five children. After the dictator was shot by partisans and hanged by the heels along with Claretta Petacci, his best-known mistress, his destitute widow returned to her native Forli. There she battled successfully for her right to a government pension, the Christian burial of Mussolini's remains, and the return of many former possessions. She also ran a restaurant-inn for 15 years. Said she: "With all the troubles in my life, if I couldn't make a plate of tortellini or bring somebody a glass of wine, I'd have jumped out the window long ago."

November in My Soul

Each November I think of a line from *Moby Dick:* "When . . . it's a damp drizzly November in my soul . . . it requires a strong moral principle to prevent me from deliberately stepping into the street and methodically knocking people's hats off." So if your soul is damp and drizzly from November on, you may have what doctors call SAD (Seasonal Affective Disorder). You can brighten your outlook with light therapy by using Vita-Lites, a special kind of fluorescent light with a spectrum that approximates summer sunlight. Psychobiologists find they can relieve clinical depressions by switching on a bright, shining light for three hours before dawn and three hours in the afternoon by tricking the brain into thinking winter is summer. (Vita-Lites are available in hardware and natural foods stores.)

GET AN ANSWERING MACHINE FOR SERENITY

If you're a working woman bombarded with phones and people and problems all day, get an answering machine. No, not for your office (or wherever you work), but for your home. Let it be your secretary. Your machine can pick up calls at home while you rest, or screen calls so you answer only those you want to deal with at the moment. Call back on the others when you're relaxed and ready to handle them. Or, if even the ring shatters your nerves, you can do what I do: Install phone jacks and disconnect the phone for total calm.

LET YOUR IMAGINATION GO

When I examined myself and my methods of thought, I came to the conclusion that the gift of fantasy has meant more to me than my talent for absorbing positive knowledge.

Albert Einstein

When my athletic Aunt Barbara used to see her teenage daughter Emily staring into space, she'd scream in exasperation: "My Lord, Emily.

Get up and do something. Don't just sit there daydreaming on a beautiful day like this." That was about 32 years ago before woolgathering and daydreaming (now called mental imagery) became respected by scientists, business people, and athletes. Mental imagery, a mind-influencing approach that Eastern cultures have valued for thousands of years, can lower blood pressure, improve athletic performance, affect planning, and diminish sexual inhibition (as you already know). You can use imagery to keep your body healthy, relaxed, and energized. Imagine a tape going in your head; the image is what you want to see yourself accomplishing. Say, I'm worried about missing a deadline. I rehearse mentally what my body should do to meet the deadline, and then my body follows what's happening in my head. If I want to relax, I might recall an amusing incident from my own life or from a movie or television show; if my self-esteem has hit rock bottom, I try to recall a time when an editor praised me for a great job. In general, you need to picture your problems and replace them in your head with solutions. Fantasies don't solve underlying problems, but they clear your head so you become more effective.

The first step is to learn to relax your body using a systematic method. The next step is to visualize your body in a healthy state. Through continued input of positive images, you can influence the circulation, nourishment, and relaxation of your body and mind.

Evoke visual images of something you enjoy looking at. Twice a day for one minute, practice imagining this favorite object, person, place, or situation.

LISTEN TO YOUR BODY

Tune in. Your body tells you when it's being pushed to the wall. Your aching back or head urges you to slow down. If you pay attention, you'll know when you need to set aside time for yourself. Aileen Crow says we should be conscious of our surroundings at all times and "consult ourselves." Are you all right? What do you want? "There's a lot of information inside when you start going for it," she says. "Your body and mind will do better if you have something to look forward to. Manufacture it if necessary. It's easy to create catastrophes—real possibilities of nuclear fallout, acid rain, terrorism—so why can't you make good things happen? Look at what is instead of what might be. We're afraid to listen to our bodies for fear of getting bad news."

A SMALL CHANGE

My friend, Leslie Cowne, a New York City therapist, endorses change. "A change is as good as a rest," she says. She means variety is the spice of life and small, frequent breaks can be as beneficial in the long run as lengthy vacations—maybe even more beneficial.

If you recall, I opened this chapter confessing the raw state of my nerves due to the Christmas season. In the days following Christmas, what should appear in the *New York Times* but an editorial, "Ranking Christmas on the Stress Scale." The writer, Joan Livingston, pointed out that on the Life Stress Scale, which assigns points to various experiences (being fired, 47 points; sex difficulties, 39 points), 12 points are assigned to the Christmas season. Christmas, writes Ms. Livingston, is rated as even more stressful than minor violations of the law. I was pleased to note that my nervous irritability was par for the course. As I worked on this chapter, preaching techniques to relieve stress, I practiced nearly all of them, chanting the phrase, This too shall pass. And now as we take on New Year's Eve, I feel absolutely wonderful.

MENOPAUSE: MYTHS & REALITIES

Chapter 8

I had never thought much about menopause until the day I walked down Madison Avenue and saw a tiny blue-and-white pillow with a needlepoint message on it: Fifty Is Nifty. Only then did I realize that menopause is close at my heels—maybe only two years away!—and that I knew little about it. Well, I was curious to know what lay ahead. The Change. Was it so dreadful? Would I lose my femininity and energy? Would I shrivel up into a little old thing? Would I lose my looks? Would I gain weight? Would I sink into depression? In the year that followed, I read everything I could lay my hands on about menopause. And I made a pest of myself asking friends who had been through menopause about their experiences and my friends on the brink of 50 about their expectations.

As I set about my reading and inquiring, I realized that most of us crowding 50 were about to enter menopause as we did menstruation—in the dark. Either that or we were bound to negative myths about menopause. "Everything suddenly sags, doesn't it?" said my 47-year-old friend Molly.

Happily, in talking to women who had gone through menopause, I found that it was a perfectly natural transition in a woman's life—you don't hit the dark bottom of despair or shrivel up. After menopause, life does go on! "Menopause is a normal change, not a tragedy, not an immense challenge, not a bad joke—just a change," writes Louisa Rose, editor of *The Menopause Book* (New York: Hawthorn Books, 1977). "How well informed you are about menopause will largely determine how well you handle it and its aftermath."

Marjorie, 50 years old, had expected the worst:

> I thought it might make me crazy because that's what I'd read in a dozen novels when I was growing up. And I'd heard about people who've gotten up drenched in the middle of the night and changed their sheets and washed their hair. I've heard of that, but it certainly never happened to me or to anyone I know.

When I spoke to my gynecologist Dr. Niels Lauersen, he told me that he is well aware of the myths about female menopause. Negative descriptions of "the change" are passed down through generations, he told me, and it's about time someone began to demystify the myths. The truth is, he said, proper nutrition, exercise, and a healthy, positive mental attitude can help women overcome the usually minor change-of-life difficulties, and even eliminate them. The late anthropologist Margaret Mead went even further: *"The most creative force in the world is a menopausal woman with zest."*

Actually as I talked with more and more women, I found out that most of them do go through menopause without going mad. In fact, a lot of my friends seemed to feel that menopause was liberating—no more birth control, no more cramps, no more pads, no more PMS. As Elaine, a 51-year-old editor/writer for a shelter magazine, said: "It was wonderful for me to stop menstruating because I had awful premenstrual tension. To stop having periods put me on an even keel. Really, menopause improved my life."

Women like Elaine have moved through "the change" without much *sturm und drang.* What I learned is that menopause, as Louisa Rose says, is not an illness or a bad joke. Neither is it a misfortune or disability. It's just another phase of life—a movement into a different age—and as the quote I recently cut from a magazine and taped over my desk says, "Every age of life has its own charms."

Menopause, the permanent end of menstruation, is a natural body change that usually takes place in women between the ages of 48 and 52, when because of a gradual decline in the function of the ovaries (starting at age 25), menstrual periods become scantier, shorter, further apart, eventually cease, and fertility ends. Although the estrogen level is too low to maintain the menstrual cycle, smaller quantities are still produced in the ovaries and the adrenal glands. But since an egg is still released occasionally, contraception (if you don't want to get pregnant) is *very* important for at least one year after your last period.

Most of us are likely to begin menopause at the ages our mothers began, but for some women menopause begins sooner, the late thirties or anytime thereafter. Other women undergo an early surgical menopause as a result of the removal of their ovaries. One type of hysterectomy removes the uterus but leaves the ovaries intact, though it ends the menstrual cycle and fertility. However, since the ovaries continue to produce hormones and eggs, this hysterectomy does not bring on menopausal symptoms.

The three most common menopausal symptoms linked to declining estrogen levels are unpredictable periods, "hot flashes," and for some women, thinning and drying of the vaginal walls. Most women experience at least mild degrees of discomfort during menopause, but there is no way to predict how much discomfort or what kind will occur in any particular woman.

THE TRUTH ABOUT HOT FLASHES

Hot flashes may take place for a few weeks or continue for years. In most cases they stop within a year or two. But while women are going through them, it's what they talk about the most. My friend Linda, 48, who talks about them a lot, says: "Having a hot flash is like suddenly experiencing the hottest day in summer even when there's snow on the ground."

"The first thing to know about hot flashes is that they are harmless," says Rosetta Reitz in her book *Menopause: A Positive Approach* (Radnor, Pa.: Chilton Book Company, 1977). "They pass quickly and are nothing to be afraid of." Hot flashes are a very common accompaniment to menopause. So common, in fact, that next to menstrual irregularities, hot flashes top the menopausal symptom list for 80 percent of all women. They are caused by an instability in the blood vessels that results from biochemical shifts in the brain. Rosetta Reitz describes a flash or flush (the two terms are used interchangeably) as "a blush only more so; the redness is deeper and the heat is hotter. It's as if the room suddenly became 20 degrees warmer and you're the only one who's noticed. But by the time you make up your mind to throw open a window, it's passed—gone in less than two minutes." Or, as my friend Linda says, it feels like a sudden burst of summer.

Busy and physically active women like Wendy, 52, an actress, have learned to deal with their hot flashes. They don't make a big deal of it. She told me that she's made peace with her flashes: "When I feel them coming on, I relax, flow with them, and breathe deeply. I become an observer of them rather than their victim."

Elaine, now 52, says:

I had my first flushed feeling on my 47th birthday. I found these flashes to be more annoying than anything else. But they never stopped me from doing anything. Although I did notice that if I was under stress or in a hot place or in the middle of a heated conversation, they would come on more frequently. It was the excitement. I used to be embarrassed about these flashes, but then I began to think of them as normal, like menstruation or pregnancy. I tried to keep in mind that they would stop, and they did just short of my 50th birthday.

Sarah, 53, says:

I know some people are embarrassed by hot flashes and never talk about them, but I think it's better to say something. There's no reason to pretend they aren't happening.

Jane, 50, says:

I take deep breaths and exhale deeply. And I've realized that exercising helps me cope, so I now exercise on a regular basis instead of sporadically. I walk about 40 minutes a day back and forth from work, and I swim or bicycle three times a week.

Edith, 48, says:

I try to avoid stress and control worry as much as I can. I think worrying brings on hot flashes.

And Susan, 53, says:

I've noticed that highly seasoned, spicy foods, coffee, tea, and alcohol trigger my hot flashes, so I stay away from them.

Some women claim that vitamin and mineral supplements have helped them with discomfort from hot flashes. Rosetta Reitz has her own nutritional formula to ban the flashes. She says that she has seen flashes disappear completely when vitamin E (no more than 800 I.U. a day) is accompanied by 2,000 to 3,000 milligrams of vitamin C, broken into smaller amounts that are taken at intervals through the day. (However, 1,000 milligrams of vitamin C is considered more reasonable by doctors.) Reitz also recommends 1,000 milligrams (also at intervals) of calcium from dolomite or bone meal. (On the other hand, some experts do *not* recommend bone meal. Calcium gluconate or calcium carbonate are preferred alternatives.)

Estrogen replacement therapy (ERT) will no doubt rid a woman of hot flashes quicker than anything else. But on the evidence, it's better to suffer the embarrassment and discomfort of the flashes than to take the risk that comes with estrogen. Scientific studies indicate that the normal risk of endometrial cancer in postmenopausal women is 1 per 1,000 per year; with regular estrogen use, the risk grows to 8 per 1,000 per year. And after prolonged use of ERT (over seven years), the risk increases 14-fold. Another hormone, progesterone, added to estrogen also relieves hot flashes and *appears* to minimize the risks (see Estrogen Replacement Therapy: The Pros and Cons, page 229). Many of the women I talked to about estrogen—and all were aware of the risks involved—tried to deal with hot flashes in other ways.

Elaine, who used estrogen for a short time and then turned to food supplements, says:

> Estrogen? I took it for a while and it controlled the hot flashes instantly, but it gave me two or three migraine headaches a week. I'm sensitive to estrogen. I never had migraines in my life until I started taking the birth control pill. I stopped it because of the migraines. Even the lowest dose of Premarin gave me a migraine that would last 36 hours. Now I handle my hot flashes with a combination of supplements and a positive outlook, which includes accepting myself. I have learned three things to let go of: judgments, comparisons, and the need to know why. I go with the flow as much as I can.

"Whether hot flashes are disabling or detrimental to the quality of life depends on many factors," says psychiatrist Anne M. Seiden, M.D., chairperson of psychiatry at Cook County Hospital in Chicago. She believes that educating women about what to expect during menopause would go a long way toward lowering their anxiety in the same way that natural childbirth classes reassure pregnant women about labor (see Menopause Self-Help Groups on page 231). As for vaginal dryness, which causes discomfort during sexual intercourse, the best remedy is lots of sexual activity or applications of lubricants such as vegetable oil, K-Y Jelly, or cocoa butter.

MORE MYTHS ABOUT MENOPAUSE

There are so many myths about menopause. One of the big ones, of course, is that you put on a ton of weight. As my 50-year-old friend Margie told me when we met for lunch after her checkup at the doctor:

> I asked my doctor if menopause would make me gain weight because so many of my friends say they're getting thick waists. My doctor looked at me through narrowed eyes and said, "*Food* makes you gain weight."

Sleep loss is another menopausal myth. Does the age 50 indeed bring on years of tossing and turning? It does seem that both men and women experience changes in sleep patterns somewhere in the middle of life. But nighttime hot flashes seem to have a minimal effect on sleep.

Meredith, 52, told me that while it was true that she woke several times a night for a few months, the hot flashes disappeared after that and her sleep pattern returned to what it had been.

At first I wasn't even aware that hot flashes had awakened me. I was so groggy when I woke up that I would go into the bathroom, have a drink of water, and go back to sleep pretty quickly. I never woke up drenched or anything like that. It was an annoyance that lasted a short time. I still went on with my regular routine during the day because I was only up for a few minutes.

And what about sex? The decline of sexual desire is yet another myth about menopause. Several friends who hadn't been through menopause yet wondered—as I did—whether your sex life flopped at the first hot flash. According to Jane Brody, who writes the syndicated "Personal Health" column for the *New York Times*:

> Sexual response is determined more by psychological than physical factors. If you think menopause marks the beginning of rapid physical deterioration, you may be more likely to let yourself go and become fat and flabby or dress unattractively even though good eating and exercise habits and attention to your appearance can help to keep you looking younger than your years. If you expect your creativity to suffer or your energy to flag, you may then stagnate, despite the fact that many women have made their greatest contributions after age 50.

Aside from possible physical discomfort, Ms. Brody says there is nothing about menopause itself that should disrupt a woman's sexual desire or activity since estrogen, the ovaries, and the uterus have no direct effect on libido. While *some* women experience a decrease in sexual desire after menopause, others become *more* interested in sex, and many are not affected one way or another. Researchers have found that the best way to continue to be sexually "capable" is to continue having lots of good sex *in* menopause, *after* menopause, and even after *that*. Fifty-three-year-old Rhoda, an attorney just married for the second time, proves Jane Brody's point that the quality of the sex does not necessarily diminish and for some it improves:

> Actually, sex is so much better since I stopped having to worry about birth control—what I would use, what he would use—and if it would really work.

Well, what about the well-known menopausal depression, where women start snarling and crying uncontrollably, or "going mad" as Elaine expected would happen? Here again, some women do experience mood changes, but the women I talked with suggested that these changes are due to corresponding family and personal changes during these years rather than a depletion of estrogen. Elaine speaks for many women:

> The truth is that I do feel low sometimes and I do feel stressed, but there is very real stress in the world today and you don't have to be menopausal to feel it. Also, do you remember when you were in your teens and you thought the world would end if the right boy didn't call you or you didn't get into the college of your choice? Do you remember the scourge of acne? Menopause seems like nothing after that.

In fact, Maggie Scarf reports in *Unfinished Business: Pressure Points in the Lives of Women* (New York: Doubleday & Company, 1980), her book on women and depression, that hospitalizations for depression and suicides occur no more often during menopause than at any other age in a woman's life. Ms. Scarf describes the research used by Dr. Myrna W. Weissman, director of the Yale Depression Unit. Dr. Weissman divided 157 depressed female patients in the outpatient department into three separate age groups—younger than 45, between 45 and 55, and 56 and over. Dr. Weissman found no differences in the severity of depressive symptoms among the women in the three age groups. As for the much-touted depression over loss of fertility, by menopause most women feel the way Elaine does. Delighted to be rid of possible pregnancy, she says, "Four children are quite enough."

As a result of my woman-to-woman research (as well as my reading), I have laid to rest for myself, and I hope for you, many of the menopausal myths. "Hot flashes" are rarely more than a nuisance; sex life can go on and with zest; weight gain happens if you overeat and underexercise; sleep patterns change as one grows older (but not because of hot flashes); and estrogen replacement therapy is more likely to harm you than to keep you forever young.

The facts are that menopause is easier to go through if you eat well, exercise vigorously and regularly, and become involved—if you're not already—with an interest or, better yet, a passion for something or someone.

Footnote: After I ended my menopausal inquiries, breathing a sigh of relief in the knowledge that neither you nor I will cave in at 50, I went back to the pillow store to buy the "Fifty Is Nifty" pillow for a friend on the verge of 50. What did I see when I got to the store but another pillow with a more inspiring—and now believable—message: "Sixty Is Sexy."

ESTROGEN REPLACEMENT THERAPY: THE PROS AND CONS

While many women have been on estrogen replacement therapy (ERT) since the 1930s, its popularity soared after 1966 when gynecologist Robert A. Wilson, M.D., who had administered estrogen to more than 5,000 women for menopause ("curable deficiency disease"), published *Feminine Forever* (New York: M. Evans & Company). Dr. Wilson advised prolonged routine ERT therapy to keep a woman looking and feeling young.

Years later, Barbara Seaman, author (with Gideon Seaman, M.D.) of *Women and the Crisis in Sex Hormones* (New York: Rawson Associates, 1977) admitted in her book that estrogen was effective in controlling hot flashes. But to Wilson's claim that "at 50 women on ERT still look attractive in sleeveless dresses or tennis shorts," Ms. Seaman replied, "True enough, some do. But so do some older women not on ERT. We think that tennis is a more likely factor."

Despite the possible side effects (edema, increased body weight, and allergic rash), women seized upon ERT as a so-called youth pill, and ERT became big business for the drug companies and the doctors who prescribed it for their patients. After the publication of *Feminine Forever,* the use of estrogen nearly tripled.

Then, in 1975, the first of eight retrospective studies linking the use of estrogen in menopause to endometrial cancer appeared. By 1977, the U.S. Food and Drug Administration (FDA) required package inserts, which advised using estrogen only for the relief of debilitating hot flashes and vaginal dryness—and then only in the lowest dosage possible and for the shortest period of time.

Evidence against using ERT began to mount. Saul Gusberg, M.D., head of obstetrics at New York's Mount Sinai School of Medicine, said he had a "morbid fear of giving women uterine cancer" through estrogen supplements.

Eight retrospective studies since 1975 have shown that the incidence of endometrial cancer in women being treated with ERT increases four- to eight-fold after two to four years of treatment, compared with the incidence in women not being treated with estrogen. "Estrogen is not a carcinogenic initiator, but a promotional agent," explains professor Barbara S. Hulka, M.D., Department of Epidemiology, School of Public Health, at the University of North Carolina. "In women who are predisposed to endometrial cancer for whatever reasons, estrogen acts as a triggering mechanism, setting the next part of the process in motion, and it acts very rapidly. The duration of use is the single most important predictor of increased risk. Estrogen use of four years or more primarily increases the risk of the early stage, which has the best prognosis," notes Dr. Hulka.

Most experts agree that too many hormones were prescribed in doses that were *too* high for *too* long. Niels H. Lauersen, M.D., gynecologist and author (with Eileen Stukane) of *PMS—Premenstrual Syndrome and You* (New York: Simon & Schuster, 1983) and *Listen to Your Body* (New York: Berkley Publishing Corporation, 1983) adds, "At a time when almost every woman with menopause was given ERT, reports began to emerge that some women who were on very high amounts of estrogen for years without pause developed endometrial cancer."

In an attempt to counteract the increased risk of endometrial cancer, another hormone, progestin, has been used as a supplement for several days of each treatment cycle. But do progestins added to the cycle diminish the risk? Although the latest research has found that the chance of cancer will be particularly low if progestin is added during the last ten days of each ERT cycle, the final results are not in yet, according to endocrinologist Dr. Stanley G. Korenman, chief of medical services at the Veterans Administration Hospital, Sepulveda, California.

In any case, both Dr. Gusberg and Dr. Lauersen advise an annual biopsy or suction curettage to monitor women on prolonged estrogen use. "It is important that the estrogen and progesterone be given under the careful supervision of an informed physician," says Dr. Lauersen. "A hormone replacement should still only be considered when a woman has severe problems with vaginal dryness, hot flashes, hot flushes, osteoporosis, or other symptoms of menopause. If ERT becomes necessary, a woman should be placed on the lowest dose of hormones that will control her symptoms. And the natural approach to symptom relief—proper nutrition, regular exercise, and vitamin supplementation—should always be tried first."

Diana Siegal, member of the Boston Women's Health Collective and a spokesperson against estrogen because of its link to breast and endometrial cancer, says that women should be wary of using ERT. "This must be of special concern to midlife women since three out of four breast cancers occur after age 50 and the peak period for breast cancer coincides with menopause," says Ms. Siegal. "Besides, ERT interferes with, covers up, distorts, and delays the body's natural adjustment to decreased estrogen levels. Most women can pass through this transition without major difficulty."

Other experts think that ERT may be used after a hysterectomy, when hot flashes can cause sudden—and often severe—discomfort. Professor Ann Voda, R.N., Ph.D., director of nursing physiology at the University of Utah's College of Nursing and author (with James Tucker) of *Menopause Me and You: A Personal Handbook for Women* (Salt Lake City: University of Utah College of Nursing, 1984) says, "I personally wouldn't take estrogen unless I had had a surgical menopause and then it becomes a viable option."

If you *can't* live with your symptoms and you and your doctor agree that ERT would be beneficial despite the risks, you should observe the following precautions:

✔ If your doctor gives you a prescription for treatment of menopausal symptoms, find out what it is and what are its possible side effects. Your doctor should take a careful history and do a thorough physical examination, including a Pap smear. If you have a family history of cancer, recurrent cysts or blood clots, had kidney or liver disease, enlargement of the lining of the uterus and endometrium, or fibroids, don't even start ERT.

✔ Make sure your doctor explains the risks of the treatment as well as the benefits. If your doctor does not seem cautious with this potentially dangerous treatment, seek the opinion of another doctor.

✔ While estrogen creams may relieve vaginal discomfort during intercourse, this form of estrogen can still be absorbed into your system (and your partner's) and its long-term effects on the body are not known.

✔ The cyclic method of taking estrogen is currently favored. This means that the woman takes estrogen for a 20- to 25-day cycle, then stops taking it for 5 to 7 days. This will help avoid possibly harmful effects of a prolonged, uninterrupted use of ERT. If more than a year goes by and your doctor has not suggested a trial period without medication, you should suggest it.

✔ Take ERT in pill form rather than in weekly or monthly injections. Side effects that can occur with ERT last longer with injections.

✔ During ERT, periodic examinations are necessary to check on the effects of the drug, to decide whether the dosage should be changed, and to evaluate the need for continuing therapy. You should take the smallest effective dose over the shortest practical period of treatment.

MENOPAUSE SELF-HELP GROUPS

Many women agree with Dr. Seiden that educating women about what to expect during menopause would help to lower anxiety about it. To that end, menopause self-help groups are springing up all over the country. As Kathleen I. MacPherson writes in *Sojourner,* the newspaper of the Menopause Collective, "Menopause self-help groups can help all of us, young and old, to understand and appreciate our menopausal

(continued on page 234)

Breast Self-Exam

Although there is no sure way to know that you will never get breast cancer, you can act to protect yourself by undergoing mammography once a year if you are past the age of 50 or at intervals determined by a physician, by cutting down the fat in your diet, and by examining yourself once a month for suspicious lumps (which usually turn out to be benign). The American Institute for Cancer Research advises that you examine your breasts one week after your period, when the breasts are usually not tender or swollen. After menopause, or if you have had a hysterectomy, examine them on the first day of each month. Follow these procedures:

✔ **Examine your breasts lying down.**
Stretch out flat on your back with your left arm behind your head. Put a folded towel under the left shoulder. Use the flat of the fingers of your right hand. Start at the base of your breast and make a series of

circular motions working in toward the nipple until the entire breast has been examined. Press firmly and deeply and take your time. Also feel the area between the breast and armpit as well as the armpit itself. Repeat the process to examine the right breast using your left hand. Finally, squeeze the nipple of each breast between the thumb and first finger. If any liquid, clear or bloody, appears, it should be reported to a doctor immediately.

✔ **Examine your breasts in front of a mirror.**
Stand in front of a mirror with your arms at your sides. Look for any irregularity in

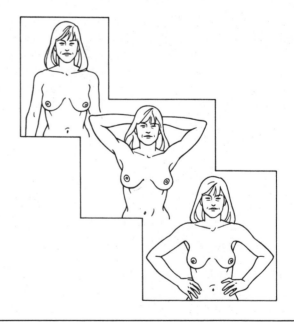

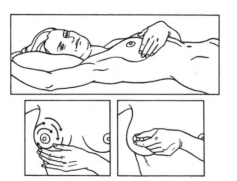

the shape of your breasts, as well as for puckering or dimpling of the skin. Repeat this inspection with your hands clasped behind your head. Then, with your hands pressed firmly on your hips, elbows out, check again for any irregularities.

✔ **Examine your breasts in the shower.** You may also find it easier to examine your breasts during a bath or shower as your hands will move easier over wet skin. Simply keep your fingers flat and move them over every part of each breast as described above.

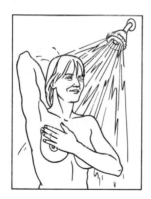

✔ **If you find a lump, dimple discharge, or thickening.**
If you find a lump, dimple discharge, or any thickening of breast tissue, do not be frightened. It probably is not cancer (eight out of ten lumps are *not*). However, only a doctor can help you to be sure. It would be wise to see your doctor as quickly as possible.

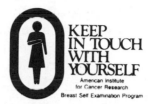

KEEP
IN TOUCH
WITH
YOURSELF
American Institute
for Cancer Research
Breast Self Examination Program

If you would like further information and/or peel-off reminder stickers (Keep in Touch with Yourself) to place inside medicine cabinets or showers or to post on calendars, write to Joanna Ramwell, Information Coordinator, BSE Department, American Institute for Cancer Research, Washington, DC 20069.

experiences as a natural and vital part of our lives." These groups, Ms. MacPherson goes on to say, are a special form of consciousness-raising that grew out of the feminist movement as women realized that control over their bodies and health care are major feminist issues.

Menopause self-help groups have been formed by the San Francisco Women's Health Center, the Berkeley Women's Health Collective, the Women's Community Health Center in Cambridge, Massachusetts, and the Santa Fe Health Education Project. (Fees vary from none to nominal for five three-hour sessions.)

If you don't have a women's health group where you live, you might want to start your own menopause support group. Here's what the Santa Fe Health Education Project advises:

First, find interested women in your community. Begin with a small number (four to seven) of women: women who have already gone through menopause and are willing to talk about it; women who are going through menopause now; and women who are interested in educating themselves even though they are not near menopause age.

Second, consider the points to be covered at the first meeting. What do people want to know? The subjects covered might include: the physiology of menopause, treatments for menopausal symptoms, feelings about menopause, and general health during the middle years. Also, discuss how to get this information and the possibility of asking speakers, doctors, and nurses to attend some meetings. Discuss what to read, experiences to share, and when, where, and for how long to meet. (The Santa Fe groups met in members' homes two hours each week for a total of five weeks.)

OUTLINE FOR DISCUSSION

Session I: General Discussion

The Santa Fe Health Education Project suggests using the following questionnaire to stimulate discussion. (There are no right or wrong answers.)

1. What is menopause?

2. Where did you first find out about menopause?

3. Have you already started or gone through menopause?

4. What are the symptoms of menopause?

5. What feelings do you have about menopause?

6. Does your family know about menopause?

7. What would you like to know about menopause?

8. If you are going through menopause now, did you use estrogen replacement therapy or other therapies?

Session II: Physiology of Menopause

Talk about the menopause books in your local library. If they are out-of-date, ask the librarian to order some newer ones. (Most librarians welcome suggestions.) In talking about the physiology of menopause, discuss menstruation. Describe an average 28-day cycle and the symptoms of menstruation. The assignment for the next session might be to read "The Crisis Couples Face at Forty" by Gail Sheehy (*Reader's Digest*, March 1977).

Session III: Treatments for Menopause

Discuss Sheehy's article. What is the central theme? (Women turning outward and away from the family and men turning inward toward the family.) Someone might ask the group, "Have you ever felt this way?" Have a discussion of treatments: ERT, tranquilizers, and natural remedies. The assignment for the next meeting might be: Try to find out more information about these therapies. Ask doctors, nurses, or talk to friends.

Session IV: Hysterectomy and Preventive Care

Discuss what each woman found out about: contraception and hysterectomy; preventive care, such as a breast self-exam; and the importance of Pap smears in detecting cancer of the cervix.

Session V: Conclusions

Conclude with a general discussion of menopause. What was learned? Discuss subjects for further study and ways to start other groups.

PREVENTING OSTEOPOROSIS

Osteoporosis (which literally means porous bone) is the loss of bone mass that weakens the skeleton and can result in spontaneous fractures or the condition that causes "shrinkage" and "dowager's hump" in women past menopause. This condition is a major public health problem that affects 15 to 20 million Americans. Osteoporosis is responsible for at least three-quarters of the more than two million bone fractures a year among American women aged 45 or older. There are about 40,000 American women who die each year in the United States from complications of osteoporosis, and it cripples many more.

At the National Institutes of Health Consensus Development Conference on osteoporosis in April 1974, experts in the field agreed that women are at higher risk than men in that they have less bone mass, and, for several years following natural or induced menopause, the rate of bone mass decline is accelerated.

White women are at higher risk for osteoporosis than black women; white men are at higher risk than black men. Women who are underweight are at higher risk for osteoporosis than overweight women. Women who have had early surgical menopause are at high risk. Women who smoke, diet, or who lead sedentary lives are at high risk. It seems many of us fit in someplace.

Even so, a lot can be done right now to overcome it by means of diet high in calcium-rich foods, calcium supplements, weight-bearing exercises such as walking and running—and, as a last resort, estrogen. Some experts say that reliable scientific studies have shown that supplementary estrogen, when started shortly after the onset of menopause, will reduce the risk of osteoporosis. However, says gynecologist Robert W. Cali, M.D. of the Lahey Clinic, Burlington, Massachusetts, "Its use remains controversial. Estrogen carries a small risk of a woman developing endometrial cancer while on it."

While experts disagree on the efficacy of estrogen supplements to forestall osteoporosis, virtually all agree on the importance of calcium and exercise to slow the rate of bone breakdown. "Bone is a living structure much like muscle, skin, or even the heart," says Daniel W. Bienkowski, M.D., of Lahey's Department of Orthopedic Surgery. "It is constantly growing and remodeling."

Robert P. Heaney, M.D., is a vice-president for the health sciences at Creighton University, Omaha, Nebraska, and a member of the American Society for Bone and Mineral Research (this group of 800 members includes specialists in organic chemistry, radiology, orthopedics, dentistry, nutrition, endocrinology, surgery, and pediatrics). Dr. Heaney outlines the guidelines of the society for the treatment and prevention of osteoporosis:

✔ Weight-bearing exercises, such as walking or playing tennis, should be a regular component of daily activity throughout life.

✔ Adequate attention to dietary calcium should be emphasized throughout life. Women who do not take estrogen replacement therapy after menopause should consume 1,000 to 1,500 milligrams of calcium daily. If adequate dietary levels cannot be met by foods alone, a daily calcium supplement is recommended.

✔ The consumption of large amounts of vitamins A and D should be avoided unless medically indicated and specifically prescribed by a physician.

✔ Cigarette smoking should be avoided.

✔ The potential use of estrogen replacement therapy following menopause should be evaluated on a case-by-case basis with one's physician.

Dr. Morris Notelovitz, gynecologist, climacteric specialist, and author (with Marsha Ware) of *Stand Tall! The Informed Woman's Guide to Preventing Osteoporosis* (Gainesville, Florida: Triad Publishing Company, 1982) and the president and founder/director of the Center for Climacteric Studies, a private, nonprofit midlife research corporation, elaborates on the rules of the Society for the treatment and prevention of osteoporosis:

✔ **Stop losing calcium!**
Too much meat, especially beef and pork, which are very high in phosphorus, can cause calcium to leach from your bones at the time when you need calcium the most. Antacids with aluminum can contribute to a "negative calcium balance."

Cutting down on coffee consumption may help. Studies show that women past menopause who drank more than four cups of coffee a day displayed signs of bone weakening more frequently than those who drank fewer than four cups.

Alcohol too is associated with decreased intestinal absorption of calcium. While alcoholics are known to be at a high risk of osteoporosis, it is not yet known exactly how much risk moderate drinking involves. If you're going through menopause, you should consider the risks of osteoporosis against your desire for alcohol.

Avoid table salt and so-called convenience foods—in general, these foods are high in salt and low in calcium. It's important to know that if you increase fiber in your diet to avoid colon cancer, the increase in elimination also carries away calcium. Fruit and vegetable fibers are preferable to cereal fibers, which are likely to increase calcium depletion.

✔ **Eat more calcium-rich foods.**
The top calcium foods, according to the U.S. Department of Agriculture *(Composition of Foods,* Agriculture Handbook No. 8, Washington, D.C.: Agricultural Research Service) are skim milk, low-fat yogurt, powdered milk, canned sardines, salmon (including the bones), and hard cheeses. Other good sources include: dried beans, broccoli, kale, and dandelion greens.

✔ **Take calcium supplements.**
Women from 20 years old to menopause should be getting 1,000 milligrams of calcium. Women over 50, or women in and past menopause, either naturally or as a result of surgery, should consume 1,000 to 1,500 milligrams daily of calcium. Many women get less than 500 milligrams per day in their diets. Calcium supplements are confusing because some types of calcium are taken up by the body better than others. Don't evaluate a supplement by price (more expensive is not necessarily better) because many calcium supplements are overpriced. Ask your pharmacist for an inexpensive calcium carbonate preparation and ask him how many tablets you need to make up your daily requirement.

Some types of calcium on the market aren't taken up as well by the bones. These include calcium gluconate, calcium lactate, dibasic calcium phosphate, and chelated calcium. Avoid anything with aluminum in it because of the effect it can have on the bowels. Don't use calcium lactate if you don't tolerate milk well. Calcium chloride frequently irritates the stomach. Calcium gluconate only works well if taken frequently throughout the day. Avoid bone meal and dolomite because of possible contamination with heavy metals such as lead.

✔ **Be sure you get enough vitamin D.**
Vitamin D is necessary for your body to use the calcium it gets. The Recommended Dietary Allowance (RDA) is 400 units, contained in most diets.

Experts agree that weight-bearing exercises and activity reduce the risks for and aid in the treatment of osteoporosis. "The three preferred methods of prevention for osteoporosis are exercise, exercise, exercise," says Lila A. Wallis, M.D., associate clinical professor of medicine, Cornell University Medical College, Ithaca, New York.

RECOMMENDED READING

MENOPAUSE

Budoff, Penny Wise, M.D. *No More Hot Flashes and Other Good News.* New York: Putnam's, 1983.

A medical approach to treating menopause.

Boston Women's Health Book Collective. *Our Bodies Our Selves.* New York: Simon & Schuster, 1984.

A women's health care perspective.

Reitz, Rosetta. *Menopause: A Positive Approach.* New York: Penguin Books, 1977.

A book on menopause from a woman's perspective.

Rubin, Lillian B. *Women of a Certain Age.* New York: Harper and Row, 1979.

Revealing accounts of women experiencing the "midlife crisis."

Seaman, Barbara, and Gideon Seaman, M.D. *Women and the Crisis in Sex Hormones.* New York: Bantam Books, 1977.

Detailed section on the estrogen replacement therapy (ERT) controversy with alternatives.

Voda, Ann M., R.N., Ph.D., with James Tucker. *Menopause Me and You: A Personal Handbook for Women.* Salt Lake City: University of Utah, College of Nursing, 1984.

How to understand and deal with this important phase of a woman's life.

Weideger Paula. *Menstruation and Menopause.* New York: Alfred A. Knopf, 1975.

A major book on two important events in a woman's life.

OSTEOPOROSIS

Notelovitz, Morris, M.D., and Ware, Marsha. *Stand Tall, the Informed Woman's Guide to Preventing Osteoporosis.* Gainesville, Florida: Triad Publishing Company, 1982.
Understanding and preventing this crippling bone disease.

MORE INFORMATION ON WOMEN'S HEALTH

Center for Climacteric Studies
University of Florida
901 8th Ave., Suite B1
Gainesville, FL 32601

The Center publishes the journals *Midlife Wellness* and *Menopause Update.*

The Menopause Collective
1938 Massachusetts Ave.
Cambridge, MA 02138

National Dairy Council
6300 N. River Rd.
Rosemont, IL 60018

Ask for a reprint of the September-October 1982 issue (vol. 53, no. 5) of the *Dairy Council Digest* on calcium metabolism and osteoporosis.

National Women's Health Network
224 7th St. SE
Washington, DC 20003

The NWHN publishes the *Menopause Resource Guide,* which contains extensive listings of references and resources around the United States. Many books and journals on women's health are available through the NWHN.

Santa Fe Health Education Project
215 W. San Francisco St.
Santa Fe, NM 87501

Menopause: A Self-Care Manual is available in English or Spanish.

Chapter 9

FLEXING
YOUR
MENTAL MUSCLE

The other day a close friend, who is 42, said, "I'm meeting a lot of interesting women, and I wish I could get to know them better. But I don't have time to make new friends." Wrong thinking. A major study on aging has shown that women who fare best later in life are those who stay in touch with old friends while making new ones.

On the other hand, Kay, another friend, age 82, has outlived most of her friends. But she goes on to make new ones, young and old. Her energy astounds me. She also reads voraciously. Kay's range of conversation is as lively as any I know. And she's always up for something new. On the day Kay and I had lunch, the menu offered an appetizer of sea urchins. "Oh," she said, "What fun. I've never had them." And without hesitation she placed her order.

Just as we must work to keep our bodies flexible, we must tone our minds. The mind, like any muscle, will function more efficiently if used. But, unfortunately, just as we approach an age when we become most interesting, we start limiting ourselves.

It's important to keep flexible and open to new experiences, to set new goals now and reach for them: to get that long-awaited M.F.A., landscape a garden, take in a foster child, learn to swim, travel to Bora Bora, go up in a hot-air balloon; do something for fun at least once a day. Dare.

I firmly believe that keeping the mind young is as much a path to fitness and beauty as situps or a new lipstick. Even more. The mind is the most accommodating part of the body; it has untold resources and can receive and retain immeasurable amounts of information. The important thing is to stimulate the mind constantly with fresh challenges, new people, unusual experiences, and an abiding sense of curiosity.

PEOPLE: MEETING THE NEW AND KEEPING THE OLD

Never allow yourself to say, "OK, that's it. I have plenty of friends and couldn't possibly make time for any more." While old friends are irreplaceable and worth their weight in gold, meeting new people and making new friendships can be exhilarating and enlivening. But, before you can increase your circle of friends, you must be willing to open yourself up to others. As they open up to you and your mutual curiosity increases, you'll find yourself learning more about each other as you both grow.

When I asked my 82-year-old friend Kay how she continued to make so many new friends, she said, "I ask a lot of questions. I'm always curious about what makes people tick." Kay's natural curiosity ensures two very important things: One, she'll always be making new friends and renewing old ones; and two, her mind will always be challenged and exercised by all the input and information that she so warmly welcomes.

A study conducted by Dr. K. Warner Schaie, professor of human development and psychology at Penn State University, gives evidence that people who are flexible and adaptable through their lives will stay more fit mentally than those who aren't. Dr. Schaie studied a group of 2,000 adults from Seattle, Washington, whose ages ranged from 22 to 88. Over a 30-year period, he looked at as many aspects of their life-styles as he could, including their occupations, incomes, leisure activities, travel, reading habits, and even the number of people they would normally see a day. Their flexibility—or ability to cope with unfamiliar situations that made new or unexpected demands on them—was measured, and the subjects were then tested for their mental ability by answering vocabulary, math, and problem-solving questions. His findings? Flexible, active people tested better across-the-board. He said, "The people who led active lives when they were middle-aged remained stable or showed improvement in mental abilities after age 60. Those people who didn't have very stimulating lives showed a marked decline." I had the good fortune of talking with Dr. Schaie, and he told me how unfortunate it was that "instead of maintaining a variety of interests in mid-life, people start subtracting them." Women should realize, he said, that "if they stand still, they are going backward in this technological age. Because of technology you might be afraid to use a bank machine or a computer, but you must force yourself to learn. You must work against your fear and look more carefully at the reasons for your avoidance," he added.

"The probability is that most women will survive their husbands," he continued. "Yet, traditionally women leave certain things to their spouses to do. Even if they drive, for example, they will leave the driving to their husbands, or they will leave the management of money to their husbands. They should keep in mind that many women in their late mid-lives are forced to learn to be independent because they are statistically likely to outlive their spouses." In the studies, conducted with his wife, Dr. Sherry Willis, associate professor of human development at Penn State University, Dr. Schaie found that women who lose their husbands suffer not only from the loss of a loved one but from the loss of opportunities they previously had. Their circles of friends get smaller, and often economic resources are less. "We tend to be a couple-oriented society, particularly among women in mid-life and older," said Dr. Schaie. "Data suggest that women without careers are particularly vulnerable to mental decline in later life," he added.

This discussion is not intended to make you morose, but to put you on guard against settling in, limiting your life. I urge you to meet new challenges.

I know a woman of 50 who recently started her own landscaping business. I know another woman of 48 who within the last three years has adopted two Tibetan daughters, both under 5 years old. Two years ago I got my M.F.A. degree in dramatic writing, something I had wanted to do since I was in my twenties. Now I've written an original play and adapted a short story into a play. I had never attempted any of this before age 45. And I really feel I've just scratched the surface of the challenges that lie ahead.

As for increasing your circle of friends, Dr. Schaie's response echoes Kay's: "If an old friend moves away or dies, don't decide you're too old to make new friends. Find other interesting people to get to know," he says.

MENTAL EXERCISES

We do exercises to keep our bodies fit. Why should our minds be any different? And just as certain exercises are designed to maintain and improve particular parts of our bodies, there are ways to give our minds the proverbial "work-out."

Of these, the most obvious and familiar is reading. Read, read, read. Read newspapers, travel brochures, recipes, and letters—all are valuable sources of new information, and all stretch your mind. One German study of elderly people, edited by Dr. Schaie, indicated that the verbal I.Q. scores of the better-educated group rose significantly when they were tested again several years later, while the less educated group had I.Q. scores that declined over the same period. The explanation: The better educated had a well-developed habit of reading. Think of your library as a gymnasium full of equipment: Each book is the equivalent of a barbell, rowing machine, exercise mat, or jump rope for your mind. The more you use the equipment, the better shape your mind will be in.

Dr. Schaie is a great champion of mental exercise. He recommends crossword puzzles and word games like Scrabble because they require using memory and mental skills. He also thinks that "anyone who can afford a computer and doesn't buy one is foolish. Computer games offer all sorts of interesting ways to exercise your mind," he said. "Look at your leisure activities," he told me, "and make choices that exercise the mind. Rather than bingo, pick some activity that involves thoughtful behavior performance and problem solving using memory skills. Don't be a spectator. Do things that are particularly challenging."

THE BODY AND MIND CONNECTION

Staying mentally fit is not just an intellectual pursuit. Your mind's health needs much the same attention as your body's, with respect to exercise, nutrition, and rest. The other day, after many late deadlines, I woke up with my mind feeling like it was swathed in cotton batting. It took a brisk walk in the cold winter air to set everything straight again.

The key to this straightening-out process was oxygen. The more oxygen delivered to the brain, the better it will function. Aerobic exercise improves the distribution and absorption of oxygen in the body and benefits the entire system, not just the brain. Regular exercise will increase the body's total blood volume, and since oxygen is carried through the system by the red blood cells, one result will be more oxygen to the brain. It's no surprise that, according to recent studies, regular exercise can actually improve your mental functioning, particularly your short-term memory.

Much has been written about the so-called "runner's high," or the feeling of euphoria brought on by the release of endorphins in the brain. Similarly, certain types of exercises that are challenging and exciting spark the brain to release stress hormones that heighten alertness and help improve the memory. A lot depends on your attitude while exercising, whether you are elated, depressed, or terrified, but the essential ingredient is oxygen, and plenty of it.

Not all exercises are appropriate for all people, however. Dr. Schaie says, "Clearly, one has to be realistic in terms of what the body will and won't do for you, and whether the activity is physically safe. One doesn't have to start mountaineering. But you could start cross-country skiing or ice skating." Dr. Schaie is particularly fond of square dancing. "Square dancing is a good example of an activity that has aerobic value but also exercises mental skills," he said. You have to remember the sequences given by the caller and translate them into organized motor behavior. And if you think that square dancing is an old-fogy activity, note that it's being touted in chic women's magazines as a terrific way to burn calories.

MIND AND MOODS

Moods are fascinating. We often don't know what causes them to come and go or why some people are terribly moody and others are pretty steady. Moods are, however, intricately linked to the brain's ability to function. And they play an enormous part in the way we learn new things, pay attention, and remember what we have learned.

Gordon H. Bower, chairman of the Psychology Department at Stanford University, has pioneered the theory of "state dependent memory." Simply put, his study suggests that if you are in a happy mood when you learn something, you will best be able to remember it when you feel happy again. This holds true for moods of all kinds, joy, sadness, anger, fear, or depression. His study, "Mood and Memory," which was reported in the February 1981 *American Psychologist,* produced some remarkable findings. By means of hypnosis, he was able to record how well his subjects could remember sad things when they felt sad and pleasant things when they were feeling happy. "People who were sad during recall [under hypnosis] remembered about 80 percent of the material they had learned when they were sad, compared with 45 percent recall of the material they had learned when they were happy. Conversely, happy recallers remembered 78 percent of their happy list versus 46 percent of their sad list." Our brains seem to operate in a highly selective fashion, and our ability to retrieve information from our mental filing cabinets varies with our emotions.

We can't always control our moods. But we can be more aware of them and recognize that these emotional ups and downs contribute a great deal to how we think, learn, and process information. You might look at it this way. If you could manage to stay happy all the time, you'd remember and take in new information in a positive way, which would reinforce you to be even more positive. And wouldn't that be wonderful?

MAYBE THERE REALLY IS A BRAIN FOOD

How often were you coaxed to eat fish as a kid because someone said it would make you smart? Well, there may have been something to that old wives' tale after all. Scientists have found that certain foods do, in fact, contain a substance that might help curb memory loss. And, yes, Virginia, that substance is present in fish.

Choline is an important B vitamin, found not only in fish, but in meat, egg yolks, and in lecithin, a supplement widely available in natural foods stores. The brain makes a vital nerve fluid called "acetylcholine," which is needed to bridge the gap between nerve cells so that they can transmit impulses from one cell to the next. Acetylcholine is crucial for proper brain functioning, and there is also evidence that it contributes to memory formation. Over ten years ago, researchers at M.I.T. discovered that choline in a very concentrated pure form (phosphatidylcholine) has an immediate effect on the brain's capacity to make acetylcholine. This surprised many scientists because the brain is protected from variations in daily food consumption by something known as the "blood-brain barrier." In general, nothing can penetrate this barrier and go directly to the brain except powerful substances like alcohol or narcotics. However, choline, in this pure form, is absorbed directly from the circulating blood and taken up by the brain.

Ever since this discovery was made, numerous studies, including one by the National Institute of Mental Health, have been conducted on choline's effect on the memory. The emerging impression is that those who suffer from a choline deficiency are most likely to experience memory improvement when given supplementary choline. Those who get enough choline in their diets are unlikely to become geniuses no matter how much supplementary choline they take. But studies continue. And meanwhile, as far as I'm concerned, it's not going to hurt me a bit to spoon a little lecithin on my morning granola.

Just as some substances can help to improve our memories, clinical research tells us that other substances can actually impair them. Three of the most notorious threats to your brainpower are alcohol, cigarettes, and the tranquilizer Valium. Social drinkers have shown in tests that they often have sieges of poor concentration, memory, and comprehension. And, says the report published in the January 1980 *Journal of Studies on Alcohol,* the effects are cumulative; the more often one drinks alcohol, the greater the risks of memory loss. Cigarette smokers, too, appear to have trouble with their short-term memories. A team of researchers from the Department of Psychiatry of the University of Edinburgh tested the ability of smokers to match names with faces and found that habitual smokers had greater difficulty remembering names than did nonsmokers. Valium, a widely sold prescription tranquilizer, can also hamper one's memory, according to a University of Iowa study.

MNEMONICS

Mnemonic devices are familiar to all of us. Many people have difficulty remembering important phone numbers, social security numbers, or names. They use mnemonics (you'll recall this from your piano lesson days) to remember the notes of the treble clef, EGBDF: Every Good Boy Does Fine. We all have a favorite way to remember things, be it an image associated with a thought, a string around the finger, or an alphabet rhyme. I make lists and lists *and* lists. It's not unusual for me to have a list stuck to my bathroom mirror, my refrigerator, or inside my front door. I even call myself on my answering machine as a reminder to do this 'n' that. And I keep a shopping bag, into which I drop whatever I need to take with me that day—shoes to be repaired, a laundry ticket, my yogurt.

ROLE MODELS

Role models are not just for kids. You can pick one at any stage in your life. That's the person you say this about: I'd like to be just like her when I get to be her age. For me, my dear friend Kay fills the bill perfectly. She is 34 years older than I am, yet she is ageless, and her enthusiasm is boundless.

If you aren't lucky enough to know someone like Kay, pick someone you've read about or seen in the movies, or even make up someone. Ruth Gordon, who died last year at 88, was a good role model—she still is. As the *New York Times* wrote of her after her death: "Miss Gordon manifested a fearsome will and an insatiable appetite for things new. . . . She never tired of exploration or conquest." Her husband, Garson Kanin, was quoted as saying that "her great joy was hanging around young people. She was very much involved in the new stuff."

Another woman who shows a great sense of adventure about life—yes, I mean it—is Sophia Loren. In her book, *Women and Beauty* (New York: William Morrow & Company, 1984), she discusses her attitude toward mid-life, the stage that she is at now, like you and I. "We must force ourselves to learn, to acquaint ourselves with the thrill of a new challenge by trying something completely different," she says. "And sometimes we must do it for ourselves, without regard for how people around us will react. . . . After all, experience teaches us that there is a risk in every new endeavor. This is why as we mature we sometimes become reluctant to risk our reputations on something new. But if you try something and fail, you will have learned a very valuable lesson: Failure isn't so awful after all."

And she continues: "To my astonishment, the world seems to have grown larger, not smaller, as I have matured. . . . I consider myself very fortunate to be living in a time when there is always a future for a woman, no matter what her age. But it has to be said that these possibilities exist only for the woman whose mind is growing, who is always prepared to try something new."

SETTING NEW GOALS AND TAKING RISKS

A new goal does not have to be some overwhelming course of action; it can be as simple as reading a new novel or perfecting a soufflé. Whatever it may be, the idea is to always have something you are looking forward to, an aim or challenge that you hope to master. The importance of setting goals is that you attempt something brand new, and that your movement becomes forward, outward, and upward.

Recently I read about an 82-year-old grandmother from California. She had been jogging for 12 years, had run marathons, and had backpacked. She had climbed Mount Whitney, the second-highest mountain in the continental United States, 17 times. This woman's expansive spirit "jumped" right off the page.

To believe that an endeavor is beyond your potential is to shut doors. And the more doors you shut throughout your life, the fewer options you will have as you mature. I like to think that there is an infinite hallway of doors ahead of me, and, though I will never get to open all of them, I have at least realized the vastness of my choices. I would hate to look at myself one day and realize that I never did half of the things I wanted to do. I don't want to regret, but I do want always to look forward to my future.

TAKING ON NEW CHALLENGES

One of my favorite risk-taking stories is about a big-time risk taker—Betty Friedan, who took on no smaller task than leading women to liberation. In the September 1984 issue of *Ladies' Home Journal,* she describes her decision to go on a wilderness survival expedition in the North Carolina mountains with nine strangers. Why Betty Friedan? Of all people she didn't need coaxing to become a full person and widen her horizons. Her many accomplishments speak for themselves. But, as she explained, she was "suffering from a denial and dread of age that makes it hard to celebrate the milestone birthdays—50, 60, or even 30." Then she heard about a trip for people over 55 offered by Outward Bound, an adventure that promised to make physical demands of its participants. The trip included two days of shooting rapids on the Chattooga River in life jackets and hard hats and, at one point, a 24-hour survival test in which she was to manage all alone in the wilderness. She said she was glad that no one on the trip knew that she was supposed to be a tough women's leader, for on this occasion she didn't even volunteer to be a captain of the small group.

At the end of the trip, the participants were expected to scale a steep, 60-foot cliff. Betty Friedan was terrified, "afraid to move, soaked in sweat, heart pounding, mouth dry." The precipice, from where she was standing, fell "farther than one can see," and at that moment she realized what she was doing and took charge of herself. "I don't have to prove myself this way," she shouted, "get me out of here this minute!" Betty Friedan, who has blazed many a path for women of all generations, saw one that she just didn't want to go for, *and* didn't have to go for. She gave herself the freedom of choice while standing on top of that cliff, and she opted to give up (which she admitted, for her, was the hardest thing in the world for her to do). Betty Friedan became aware of her limit in that split second, and that was a moment of discovery and enlightenment, not one in the least of defeat. She had taken on a new challenge, and that in itself was a victory.

As Dr. Schaie says, our mental acumen is sharpened by newness in all things. That newness may be no more than insight we gain into ourselves that we never had before.

AVOID MIND-DEADENERS

We have all heard about the deadening effects many things can have on our minds. For example, parents the world over try to steer their children away from the "boob tube" in favor of more educational pursuits. At every age we need to sharpen our inner resources if we are to be interested in ourselves and interesting to others. Boring people can be deadening. Nurture your mental abilities by adding new people, information, and experiences to your life at every opportunity. And if the opportunities don't come along fast enough, search them out for yourself!

NEW OPPORTUNITIES AND CHALLENGES

I could never attempt to give a complete listing of all of the possible adventures available in this world. There is one around every corner. But I have come up with a beginning, which I hope will serve as a springboard for you to seek out many more opportunities and challenges on your own.

ADVENTURES

Appalachian Mountain Club
Pinkham Notch Camp
Gorham, NH 03581
(603) 466-2727

The Appalachian Mountain Club operates a chain of huts in New Hampshire's White Mountains, which makes hiking in that area not only breathtaking, but less burdensome. The huts have sleeping and eating facilities, allowing the hiker to enjoy the scenery with a light knapsack instead of tons of gear.

Heber Adirondack Holiday
(518) 793-3855

Jeff Stanton-Skylark (Ballooning)
(914) 677-5454

Wurtsboro (NY) Airport (Gliding)
(914) 888-2791

As far as thrills go, nothing beats being airborne. Whether you prefer hot-air balloons, gliding or sky-sailing, the sensation of being aloft in the clouds is great for giving you a little perspective on life down below. Most local airports offer some form of gliding or can recommend a good spot in your area.

Mountain Travel
1398 Solano Ave.
Albany, CA 94706
(415) 527-8100

These adventures include a camel safari through the Sahara Desert in southern Algeria, a trek through Peru to the Incan ruins at Machu Picchu, and a raft trip down the Tatshenshini River in Alaska. The company's lavishly illustrated 30-page catalog lists more than 250 treks, outings, and expeditions to all seven continents.

Outward Bound U.S.A.
384 Field Point Rd.
Greenwich, CT 06830
(203) 661-0795

Outward Bound can be a mind- and body-challenging experience, as Betty Friedan discovered. Expeditions are offered by the different Outward Bound schools, located in Minnesota, Oregon, North Carolina, Maine, and Colorado. The trips can include canoeing, hiking, sailing, rafting, and dog sledding. The length of the trip and price depend on the school and the activity.

Sierra Club Outings
730 Polk St.
San Francisco, CA 94109
(415) 776-2211

Year-round, the Sierra Club offers 250 to 300 outings all over the world. April through July are the months for their Nepal springtime treks. Most people on the Sierra outings are single, and great numbers of them are middle-aged. They also have service trips, which are ten days spent cleaning up wilderness trails.

Woman's Way Fitness Adventures
Box 8668
Truckee, CA 95737
(916) 587-0887

In recent years, this program has taken place in various locations, including Guadalajara, Mexico; Jackson Hole, Wyoming; and Tahoe City, California. The adventures usually last five days and include exercise classes, rafting, windsurfing, horseback riding, or canoeing. Write to them for information.

HEALTH AND FITNESS

Aspen Health Center
P.O. Box 1092
Aspen, CO 81611
(303) 925-3586

In the magnificent Colorado Rockies is a resort with complete fitness and exercise programs, classes in dance and aerobics, as well as facials, massages, saunas, and Jacuzzis.

New Age Health Farm of Neversink Ltd.
Neversink, NY 12765
(914) 985-2221

This lovely health farm is located on 106 acres on a hilltop in upstate New York. The farm offers many services from weight reduction to the restoration of health of women suffering from problems of poor nutrition and stress. The program includes nutrition, therapy, meditation, yoga, breathing techniques, biofeedback, massage, and beauty treatments.

NETWORKING

Home Exchange International (NY)
(212) 349-5340

International Home Exchange (CA)
(415) 382-0300

Vacation Exchange Club (AZ)
(602) 972-2186

There are now many organizations that deal in the business of home exchanges. These agencies make the arrangements for you to swap homes or apartments with people from abroad. It's a great way to see a new country from the vantage point of a private home, and to meet new people.

Resources for Mid-Life and Older Women
226 E. 75 St. Suite 1D
New York, NY 10010
(212) 696-5501

Resources is a nonprofit social service agency center for women over 45 and is the first of its kind in the country. It provides women with information and counseling on careers, the empty nest syndrome, money management, divorce, menopause, widowhood, etc. Classes are given on many subjects, support groups are formed for people with similar interests and needs, and more, it is a place to make new friend-ships. Fees are on a nominal sliding scale.

RELIGIOUS RETREATS

Sufi Order
Lebanon Springs, NY 12114
(518) 794-8181

Choosing a spiritual retreat is a very personal matter, and the right one for you depends entirely on what your faith is, or what faiths you're comfortable with. I do know, from my own experience at a Sufi retreat, that the opportunity to spend time contemplatively led to my making many vital realizations about who I was, what I wanted, and where I was going.

SPORTS

Jackson Ski Touring Foundation
Jackson, NH 03846
(603) 383-9355

Jackson is a marvelous site for cross-country skiing, one of the best forms of acrobic exercise. Less expensive and less dangerous than downhill skiing, cross-country skiing can be done almost anywhere there's snow. Write or call Jackson Ski Touring Foundation for informa-tion. Your local department of recreation might be able to offer a few suggestions for places near you.

National Masters News
P.O. Box 2372
Van Nuys, CA 91404
(818) 785-1895
Attention: Al Sheehan

Information and training advice about Masters events (long-distance running, track and field, and race-walking competitions and their clubs around the country) are available.

U.S. Masters Swimming Inc.
5 Piggott Lane
Avon, CT 06001
(203) 677-9464

These clubs are for people 25 and over who love to swim—everything from laps to competition. Sixty percent of the organization's members are over 40: 55 percent are men; 45 percent are women. As well as swimming, there are other social aspects to these groups—picnics, hayrides, dances, and canoe trips.

WORKSHOPS

Art New England Summer Workshops
P.O. Box 140
Chestnut Hill, MA 02167
(617) 782-4218

In the past, Vermont's Bennington College has hosted art workshops for one, two, or three weeks during the summer. Classes are given in all of the fine arts and more, from painting, drawing, and sculpture to fabric dying and papermaking. (Access to the nearby festivals at Saratoga and Tanglewood make this program extra special.)

Augusta Heritage Arts Workshop
Davis & Elkins College
Elkins, WV 26241
(304) 636-1903

This program in central West Virginia was inspired by local people concerned with preserving traditional art forms. Most of these programs (about 75 of them) run about one week, from mid-July to mid-August, and cover subjects as diverse as square dancing, quilting, log-cabin restoration, the Irish harp, and blues harmonica.

Music Making Workshop
Paul Winter Consort
Box 68
Litchfield, CT 06759
(203) 567-9720

For five days in August, you can make music with musicians (the Paul Winter Consort among them) and nonmusicians. Musicians bring instruments; nonmusicians bring a rock, a couple of spoons, and a pan to bang. They all make music together. There's also exercise, volleyball, hiking, and vegetarian food. Usually 60 people attend at a time, people of all ages, but for the most part single.

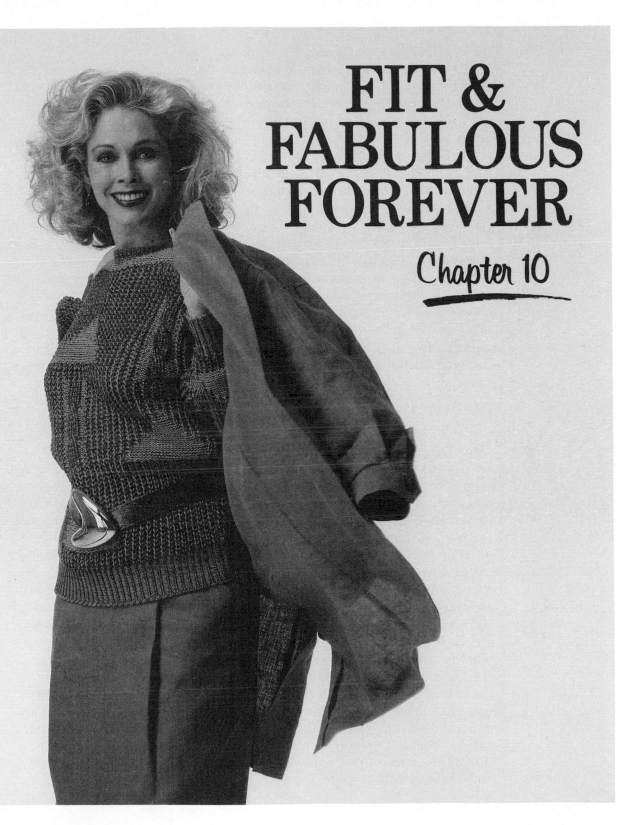

FIT & FABULOUS FOREVER

Chapter 10

Well, there you have it. We've been through scores of pages together. And by now you've got the picture. You *can* feel better. You *can* look better. You can do a lot more than you think you can. And you must!

Now I know what you're thinking. Sure, fine! But how am I ever going to find the time for all this—for the exercise and, good grief, even the time to keep a hair appointment? And the diet—I've never stuck to a diet in my life. I can't possibly do all this and take care of the rest of my life too. And do this forever—what am I, superwoman?

Well I said you were getting more than a beauty and fitness book. I promised you'd get a challenge. I know you haven't got a minute; most days I don't either. But the truth is, your schedule is more flexible than you realize. It's a matter of priorities, my dear. The foremost priority at this time of life is guess who. You.

So set up your schedule so you now focus a little more on yourself. (How's that for a change!) Don't you hear it resound in your ears right now—you're such a selfish girl! Well, all right, so be it. Now you're going to get your beauty and fitness program into your own time frame. You're no longer going to fit yourself into everybody else's schedule.

SOME TOOLS YOU'LL NEED

You'll need two inexpensive but major tools to organize yourself: a calendar (the one you have already will do) and a journal in which to enter your weight losses, energy levels, and attitudes, so you'll stay on target. I'm going to tell you how to use them to help you stay with the program you'll be designing for yourself. I'll also give you some techniques to use in avoiding those negative attitudes that come up ("What, I didn't lose a pound since yesterday—I think I'll eat a pie").

Ready. Let's go! From this day forward, you are watching what you eat, you are exercising, and you are keeping up with your grooming—which includes all those behind-the-scenes essentials: going to the cleaners, shopping for clothes, having your shoes repaired, and getting your nails done. About now I can almost hear you reminding yourself of all those things your mother or your Sunday (or Saturday) School teacher told you about vanity and self-indulgence. To stop you in your tracks from going any further with this, I want to point out that countless psychological studies show that attractive people are perceived as more intelligent, honest, stable, and friendly than others. So if you are out to prove that you're a worthwhile, intelligent person with terrific values because you don't bother with how you look, forget it. But plant this in your mind. The way you look and feel are linked to each other and the way others perceive you. In other words, you feel and look better when you feel and look better. How's that for a paradox! Just think of the times you felt your life really was going nowhere; then, you got a flattering new haircut. Remember what it did for your self-esteem? And when people told you how good you looked—well, didn't your sense of well-being hit the jackpot, and didn't your self-confidence go over the top?

Now, pardon me if I repeat myself. But you *can* look and feel good all the time (well, at least most of the time—there's always the flu). You *can* regenerate yourself. You *can* retard the aging process. You *can* go from flabby to svelte, from passive to active. It's true you can't take your face and body for granted as you did in your twenties and thirties. At this stage of your life, you have to work at looking and feeling great. You have to be careful about diet and persistent about exercise. You have to avoid the noonday sun, and you must never go out in the hot summer sun without a sunscreen. You must keep your makeup fresh and your hair in shape.

THE CALENDAR TO KEEP YOU IN LINE

Here's where your calendar helps to keep you in line. Plan one or two months ahead: Using red ink, write down the three days a week you *must* do your aerobics. Write in the days on which you do stretch

Sunday	Monday	Tuesday	Wednesday	Thursday	Friday	Saturday
		1	2 *aerobics*	3 *cleaners*	4 *aerobics*	5 *lunch - Molly 12:30 p.m.*
6	7 *aerobics*	8	9 *aerobics dinner - Harriet & Bob 7:00 p.m.*	10 *stretch*	11 *aerobics*	12
13 *brunch - Jeanne & Liz 11:00*	14 *aerobics*	15 *shoes for repair*	16 *aerobics*	17	18 *aerobics*	19 *haircut 1 p.m.*
20 *lose 2 lbs.*	21 *aerobics*	22	23 *aerobics*	24 *stretch*	25 *aerobics*	26
27 *tennis 10 a.m.*	28 *aerobics*	29	30 *aerobics*			

exercises. On Sunday write in a reminder of the two pounds you promised to lose during the week before. Ink in your once-a-month haircut.
And take these appointments as seriously as you would your time with
your dentist, your allergist, or your gynecologist.

One word of caution: When you're on your way to overhauling
yourself, it's important to avoid negative people who undermine your
efforts by harping on chronological age when it's biological age (what
shape you're actually in) that counts. "Why bother, it's all downhill from
now on," the harpies will say. When these downbeats talk piously about
"aging gracefully," they mean passively. But you have to be a participant,
not a spectator, in the way you live your life. So select positive people to
be a part of your life. Make time for friends you can laugh with and who
cheer you on. If you're so busy that you let weeks go by without calling
anyone, go through your address book and make a list of people to call,
then clip the list to the beginning of the current week in the calendar.
Then make a date with a different person each week for the next four
weeks. Mark their names in red in your calendar, along with the aerobics days and the haircut appointment—not to mention the work deadlines, the birthday present to buy for your daughter-in-law, the morning
you must let the plumber in, the dinner you must have with your
husband's boss, and on and on. Remember: This is a beauty and fitness
rule—you must ink in your own needs at the beginning of the week
before you fill in your calendar with anything else.

DEALING WITH THE DIET

Now on the theory that you *are* what you eat, let's deal with the diet.
This is an easy diet to stay with because you won't feel deprived, and the
more you stick with it, the more you will feel great surges of energy week
after week. Don't worry about getting the wilted feeling that comes with
fad diets; remember such diets are usually geared to younger women
who have more stamina than you and I do. This is a diet especially
geared to you, at your age. As you gradually become accustomed to a new
and balanced way of eating—heavy on the complex carbohydrates—
you'll less likely miss the foods that put on the pounds and deplete your
energy—cookies, cakes, and ice cream. The healthful, varied, and great-
tasting foods in the Turn-Back-the-Clock Diet (see page 19) contain the
nutrients you need to look great and function in top form. Once you are
accustomed to eating this way, once you get into the rhythm of eating
reasonable portions and of eating certain foods at certain meals, you'll
automatically know how to substitute one food for another to vary your
diet in the future.

Since I'm sure we agree that there's no point in sabotaging your initial efforts toward a healthier life, stay motivated by following these techniques: (1) Make a master shopping list for the first three weeks of the diet and clip it in your daily calendar to refer to in the following weeks. If your kitchen is stocked with only healthful foods, you won't be able to kid yourself into pigging out on jam and bread because "there is nothing else to eat." (2) Carry fruit, carrot sticks, and high-fiber crackers with you; that way you won't have the excuse to grab a hot dog when you're in too big a hurry to eat a proper meal.

The "I have no time" excuse has to go. It takes no time to decrease your intake of high fatty foods: butter, ice cream, and marbled steaks. It doesn't take time to eliminate foods high in sugar and salt, to decrease meat intake, and to increase your quota of grains, cereals, pasta, and vegetables. It means breaking with old habits and reinforcing yourself with new ones. Here again is where your journal comes in; here's how: Take a sheet of paper and head it "Ten Reasons Why I Want to Lose Weight." Then write *your* reasons, such as "It would be fun to go shopping for clothes again," or "I'll look good in a bathing suit," or "I'll be able to wear belts now." Take another sheet of paper and write down exactly "How I Would Look If I Looked My Best." Close your eyes and conjure up a picture of how you looked at your best—or how you could look at your best. Then describe the picture in your journal. Look at your journal daily to reinforce your incentive.

Ten Reasons Why I Want to Lose Weight:

1. It would be fun to go shopping for clothes again.
2. I'll look good in a bathing suit.
3. I'll be able to wear belts now.
4. My slacks will fit better.
5.

How I Would Look If I Looked My Best:

1. My hair would have the latest cut.
2. My clothes would always be pressed.
3. My shoes would always be in good repair.
4. My nails would be manicured.
5. My makeup would always be fresh.
6. My stockings would not have runs.

It's great if you can find a friend to go through your new fitness and beauty regime with you. That kind of support can help a lot. But we're not giggling teenagers any more, so it's harder to find a buddy who can fit into your schedule. However, your journal can be your buddy. Rereading your list of why you want to lose weight and your descriptions of how you looked when you looked your best are powerful spurs to action. I also clip from magazines little poems that strike my fancy and pertinent aphorisms like "Slow and Steady Wins the Race." Nothing new or glamorous in that, but the longer I live, the more I know it to be true—especially in matters of losing weight. My other great source for uplifting clippings is the obituary page in the newspaper. From Ruth Gordon's obituary, for example, I saved this life-saving logic concerning unmet schedules, "If I don't make it today, I'll come in tomorrow." In a way your journal is even better than a buddy because it focuses exclusively on you. And you can tell it *anything*. I also enter compliments, such as, "Donna, don't get any thinner. You look so good." (I forget who said that the sweetest words in the English language are "You've lost weight, haven't you?" and "I love you.")

In the journal also enter what you ate that day, when you ate it, and what your feelings were at the time. For example:

> Saturday, breakfast at 8 A.M. with Art and kids. Plain yogurt, fresh blueberries. Feeling harassed. Not especially hungry. Lunch, Evelyn, about 12:30. Starved. Ate sandwich, cheese, lettuce, cucumbers, and mushrooms on pumpernickel. "Murphy's." Dinner with Art, Julliette, and David. Roast leg of lamb, brussels sprouts, noodles, and cabbage salad with Russian dressing. Dessert, lemon meringue pie. Black coffee.

You'll see that except for the salad dressing and lemon meringue pie, you did really well on the fifth day of the diet. That will reinforce you for the following day, and you'll be careful to use lemon juice or vinegar on your salad and go without the pie.

If you pig out at your son's birthday dinner, eat less the next day. You haven't blown it, and you're not doomed to a life of fat because of occasional parties and dinners with friends and family. The great thing about this program is its flexibility.

Use your scale and calorie counter only as guidelines. If you go up a pound, don't panic. The foods you take in or omit don't register on the scale immediately. And even if you do put on a pound, don't be discouraged and drop the diet in despair. Just go easier on the calories the next day.

If weighing yourself discourages you, buy yourself a new belt—one you'd really love to wear—in a size that fits you now or even one size smaller. Drape it over a chair where you see it and try it on from time to time. You'll be thrilled when you have to punch in another notch.

Give yourself rewards. The presents don't have to be grand—buy yourself a bunch of daisies, a new sweater, or theater tickets for you and your husband when you've lost ten pounds or two inches from your thighs (one from each thigh).

Buy some Post-its, those little pads of gummed paper, and leave notes to yourself around the house, or put them in your calendar or journal to remind you to "Remember calcium supplements!"

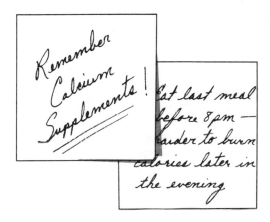

THE ESSENTIAL ELEMENT: EXERCISE

Don't think diet alone will work miracles. Diet and exercise are inexorably linked, so you'll have to incorporate exercise commitments into your calendar and your journal. The main idea is to start slowly and to be very disciplined until you get underway. You need the structure early on. Even if you start a moderate walking program, don't overdo it. Be consistent in your efforts because consistency (in the diet, as well as the exercise) is important in how you feel and in how quickly you lose weight. In other words, don't try for a marathon the first day out or you'll become discouraged by sore muscles.

This is also important—find an exercise that fits into your schedule. If your schedule is jammed, maybe getting to and from a gym or class is too much. Maybe you don't want to spend the extra minutes showering and changing. In that case, it might be wise to invest in home equipment—there's a jump rope that packs easily when you travel, or there are free weights for focusing on your arms and legs. There are rowing machines and exercycles (ones that even work the arms). There are scores of exercise tapes to use on a VCR, which offer the convenience of exercising at home with the discipline and leadership of a class. Don't miss out on your exercise if you know it's going to be an especially crowded day. Get up an hour earlier—and go to bed earlier. And if you miss an exercise session, don't beat up on yourself about it, just go on the next day. If you miss a week because you're on vacation, start again the following week. Again this is called being flexible—and it will certainly help you a lot more than being rigid would in reaching your goal.

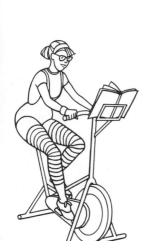

One thing you must do, and that is find an exercise that you like. Some people shrink back in horror from the very concept of exercise, but that's because they haven't found the right one for them. When you discover an exercise you really enjoy, you won't drop out; you'll look forward to it. Maybe you'd like an exercise that carries a social element with it: skating, square dancing, or tennis. Maybe you'd prefer a solitary exercise: swimming, running, or walking. Think about *where* you'd like to exercise—outdoors or indoors, on an exercycle, rowing machine, or trampoline. Decide whether you have the discipline to exercise on your own. Or consider whether you really want to spend time in an aerobics class with a crowd when you could exercise as well alone.

Even people who enjoy exercising sometimes become bored by it. If you do, use techniques to get you through it. Walking is the easiest way to start exercising, but if merely walking bores you, enlist the help of a Walkman and walk with music (never in traffic, however!). If the excitement of exercising alone at home begins to pall, watch the early morning or late evening news shows while you exercise, and the time will pass more quickly. If you buy a bookrack for your exercycle, you can read a magazine in one session or a short novel in a week. Instead of eating lunch, get together with some office co-workers and organize a lunchtime exercise program. You can also burn calories in small ways: Walk to work, walk after dinner, or walk to the market and back. Walk up the department store escalator. Climb the stairs in your apartment house or at work. And for incentive, clock your progress on a pedometer. You can buy one at any sporting goods store.

GOOD GROOMING, THE FINISHING TOUCH

Even if you're thin and trim and energetic, you're still not finished with your personal regeneration. There's grooming. Some lucky women have always known how they want to look, and they enjoy the very act of getting dressed. They go through life taking care of their clothes and themselves and make little adjustments in clothes, hair, and makeup to acknowledge the passing of time. I'm not one of them. Until recently, something was always out of kilter—a button unsewn, a shoe unshined. I've tried several looks, and finally in the last few years I found the right one for what and who I am. If you're still wavering between the ingenue you and the you of today, find a suitable role model whose hair and clothes and general look you like. Cut out pictures of how you'd like to appear and paste them up inside your closet door. Don't take Sophia Loren as your role model if you're more like Sally Field. Don't try for Joan Collins or Elizabeth Taylor either if they're far off the mark (and they probably are). A friend of mine once told her female psychotherapist she always left the beauty parlor disappointed because after all that work she still didn't look like Elizabeth Taylor. "Most of us are happy if we look better when we come out than when we went in," said the therapist.

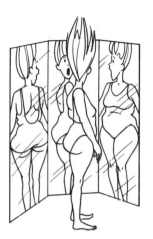

Get a full-length or even better a three-way mirror to see how you look from the back and in profile. A friend tells me she always looks good from the front because as she gets dressed, she poses with a smile. So smitten is she by her own smile that when she looks at herself in a department store three-way mirror, she's shocked to see two other sides of herself. For a similar reason hairdressers seem to do better with us than we do with ourselves; they can see the backs of our heads.

If you want to look really well turned out, you can do a lot by concentrating on your accessories. Keep your jewelry supply where you can see it as you dress, not crammed away in the back of a drawer or in a box. An immaculately dressed friend stacks her cuff bracelets over an old-fashioned hat stand. Another friend stacks hers on used hair conditioner bottles. They're very decorative and remind her to wear them. I have another friend who hangs up her scarves, beads, and small purses on a hat rack and clips her earrings onto a wire hanger. When your jewelry and purses are right in front of your eyes, you are reminded that you have many choices and you tend to take advantage of them.

Some women manage to exit from the house in the morning quickly and beautifully put together despite dealing with chaos in drawers and closets. I'm not one of them. I like organization, and I look better and dress faster when everything's in its place. If you are one of the enviable ones with a walk-in closet, you can install pegboard and see-through dividers to store jewelry and purses. Otherwise make order in a small closet and on the top and the inside of your bureau.

All this may seem awesome right now, but once you start you'll develop a rhythm—your own, of course. I don't mean that you should devote your entire life to yourself. If you work on being flexible and adaptable, you'll stay mentally as well as physically fit, and you won't lose enthusiasm for your beauty and fitness program. It's also important to remember that the more you do, the more you can do. Set and reach for new goals and open yourself up to new experiences.

When you're stretching your body, you must also stretch your mind. Don't be a spectator or ever think that life has passed you by. The challenge lies in energizing yourself and expanding your life. You can do it. I know you can. And I'm counting on you.

INDEX

Page numbers in boldfaced type indicate material in tables, captions, or boxes.